COOK YOUR BEST LIFE

MEDITERRANEAN
COOKING RECIPES

Easy Recipes for Every Day

EDITORS OF NUTIRO

© Copyright 2025 - All rights reserved.

The content contained within this book may not be reproduced, duplicated or transmitted without direct written permission from the author or the publisher.

Under no circumstances will any blame or legal responsibility be held against the publisher, or author, for any damages, reparation, or monetary loss due to the information contained within this book, either directly or indirectly.

Legal Notice:
This book is copyright protected. It is only for personal use. You cannot amend, distribute, sell, use, quote or paraphrase any part, or the content within this book, without the consent of the author or publisher.

Disclaimer Notice:
Please note the information contained within this document is for educational and entertainment purposes only. All effort has been executed to present accurate, up to date, reliable, complete information. No warranties of any kind are declared or implied. Readers acknowledge that the author is not engaged in the rendering of legal, financial, medical or professional advice. The content within this book has been derived from various sources. Please consult a licensed professional before attempting any techniques outlined in this book.

By reading this document, the reader agrees that under no circumstances is the author responsible for any losses, direct or indirect, that are incurred as a result of the use of the information contained within this document, including, but not limited to, errors, omissions, or inaccuracies.

ISBN: 978-0-9835300-7-7

Claim your free gifts!

(our way of saying thank you for your support)

Simply visit my.nutiro.com to receive:

- 30 Day Meal Plan for Cook Your Best Life Mediterranean Cooking Recipes
- Bonus companion guide of all recipe photos within each section

Hurry... both gifts are only available for a limited time

Table of Contents

Introduction 6
   What Foods Are in the Mediterranean Diet? 7
   Mediterranean Diet Shopping List 9
   Recipe Layout 11

Chapter 1: Dinner Mediterranean Style 12
   Smoked Salmon and Feta Fritters 13
   Marinated Chicken and Beef Kabobs 14
   Greek Moussaka 15
   Spanish Paella 17
   Sesame Chicken with Snap Peas and Peppers 18
   Mediterranean Gnocchi 19
   Chicken, Vegetables, and Risoni Salad 20
   Mediterranean and Basil Pasta 21
   All-In-One Fish Supper 22
   Saffron Lamb Tagine 23
   Rosemary Grilled Lamb Chops 24
   Spanish Meatball and Bean Stew 25
   Fish and Lemony Potatoes 26
   Mediterranean Marinated Tenderloin 27

Chapter 2: Lunch Mediterranean Style 28
   Grilled Tuna with Spinach and Chickpeas ... 29
   Mediterranean Marinated Flank Steak 30
   Savory Harissa Chickpea Stew Over Creamy Millet 31
   Roasted Vegetable and Quinoa Bowl 32
   Stuffed Eggplant 33
   Easy Mediterranean Pocket Sandwich 34
   Chicken Penne with Broccoli and Cheese .. 35
   Salmon and Cucumber Bowl 36
   Chicken Salad with Cilantro and Tomatoes . 37
   Greek Quinoa Bowl 38
   Spanish Frittata 39
   Chicken Quinoa Bowl 40
   Salmon Pita 41
   Greek Spanakopita 42

Chapter 3: Breakfast And Snacks 43

Breakfast Mediterranean Style 44
   Oeufs Brouillés 45
   Muffin Frittatas 46
   Mediterranean Sunkissed Granola 47
   Chickpea Hash and Eggs 48
   Fig and Ricotta Overnight Oats 49
   Mediterranean Egg Muffins 50
   Berry Chia Pudding 51
   Shakshuka 52

Snacks Mediterranean Style 53
   No Bake Coconut Cookies 54
   Salmon, Cucumber, and Avocado Bites 55
   Chocolate Cupcakes 56
   Almond Butter Mug Cake 57
   Mascarpone and Berries Toast 58
   Yogurt With Blueberries and Honey 59
   Beet Hummus 60
   Sweet and Savory Mezze Platter 61

Chapter 4: Keto-Friendly Mediterranean 62
   What is the keto diet, and how does it work? 62
   Meal Planning and Preparation 63
   Keto Breakfast Muffins 64
   Keto-Friendly Frittata 65
   Mediterranean Branzino 66
   Mediterranean Grilled Swordfish 67
   Mediterranean Chicken Salad 68
   Chicken and Pesto Zoodles 69
   Stuffed Avocados 70
   One Skillet Greek Isle Chicken 71
   Seafood Stew 72
   Tuscan Garlic Chicken 73

Chapter 5: Gluten-Friendly Mediterranean ... 74
- Meal Planning and Preparation 75
- Quinoa Salad 76
- Mediterranean Egg Bowl 77
- Gluten-Free Muffins 78
- Shrimp Zoodles 79
- Moroccan Chicken Stew 80
- Grilled Salmon Salad 81
- Polenta Pizza 82
- Quinoa and Kale Stew 83
- Caprese Pasta Salad 84
- Turkey Skillet Meal 85

Chapter 6: Vegan-Friendly Mediterranean .. 86
- Meal Planning and Preparation 87
- Broccoli and Tofu 90
- Vegan-Friendly Pilaf 91
- Mediterranean Hummus Bowl 92
- Burbara 93
- Green Olive Salad with Pomegranate Molasses 94
- Lettuce Wraps with Tahini Dressing 95
- Vegetable and Bean Salad with Basil Vinaigrette 96
- Roasted Vegetable Bowl 97
- Roasted Red Pepper Hummus with Quinoa Chickpea Salad 98
- Mediterranean Vegan Pasta 99

Chapter 7: Vegetarian-Friendly Mediterranean 100
- Meal Planning and Preparation 101
- Mozzarella Omelet 102
- Lemon Ricotta Pancakes 103
- Mediterranean Grill Tofu 104
- Greek Yogurt Parfait 105
- Orecchiette with Broccoli and Basil Sauce .. 106
- Lentil Salad 107
- Greek Salad with Hummus 108
- Veggie Wrap with Cilantro Hummus 109
- Mediterranean Quiche 110
- Baked Feta Pasta 111

Chapter 8: Paleo-Friendly Mediterranean .. 112
- Meal Planning and Preparation 113
- Zesty Mediterranean Chicken Salad 114
- Paleo-Mediterranean Frittata 115
- Zesty Lemon Bars 116
- Apple Tuna Bites 117
- Chicken Fricassee 118
- Mediterranean-Paleo Chicken Skillet 119
- Braised Cod with Leeks 120
- Meatballs and Zoodles 121
- Pork Filet with Apple Sauce 123
- Easy and Delicious Shrimp Sheet Pan 124

References 125

INTRODUCTION

Following a wholesome diet has never tasted so good! Suppose you're longing for indulgent and delicious food options that don't sacrifice flavor for a good lifestyle. In that case, you'll enjoy the over 100 recipes in this Mediterranean cookbook—from tasty appetizers to scrumptious desserts. You will satisfy any appetite with this collection of flavorful Mediterranean dishes.

From pasta primavera to fig couscous and stuffed eggplant, each recipe brings something unique and unforgettable.

The editors of Nutiro.com crafted Mediterranean recipes so that you can plunge into this cookbook and discover what to eat for breakfast, lunch, dinner, and even snacks. Even if you prefer gluten-free, keto, paleo, vegan, and vegetarian selections, you'll find delicious meals perfect for any diet.

We handpicked some of our favorite recipes from my.Nutiro.com custom meal plans and added a lot of new recipes that will transport your Mediterranean experience!

Whether making easy dinner recipes, your family will love the savory lunch options, light salads, yummy snacks, and warm breakfast dishes. This cookbook allows you to savor all the benefits of a Mediterranean diet without compromising taste or satisfaction.

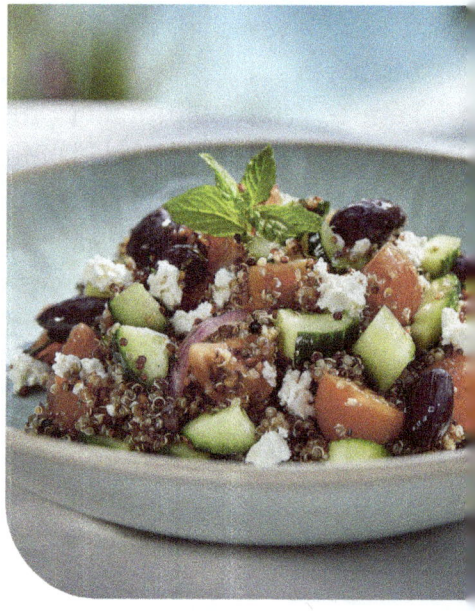

This easy-to-follow guide on what to eat will have your family asking for another serving! Your culinary adventures await—with delicious, hearty recipes inspired by the unique cuisines of the Mediterranean region, this cookbook offers an easy-to-follow approach to making healthful and flavorful meals.

Full of nutrition advice, tips on creating healthy meals that are surprisingly tasty, and guidelines for achieving long-term healthy lifestyle and wellness goals, your kitchen will become a gateway to the abundant flavors of Italy, Greece, and beyond.

Enjoy culinary traditions and inspirations from the Mediterranean region

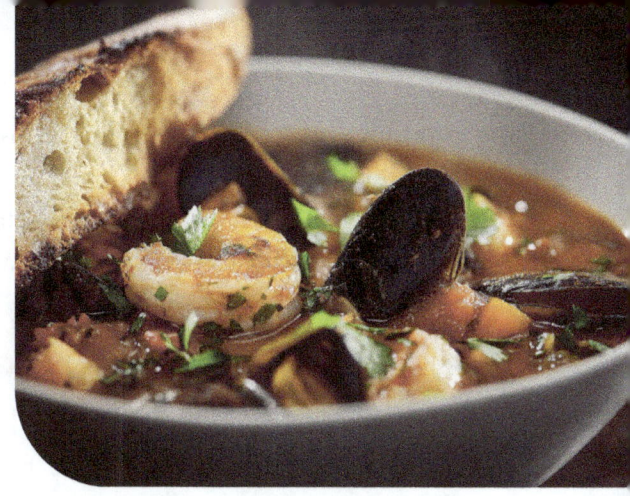

The Mediterranean region is defined as a geographical area bounded by the sea on three sides. It covers parts of Europe, North Africa, and the Middle East, extending from Spain in the west to Turkey in the east. This diverse and vibrant region has been home to many different cultures throughout history, with influences from Ancient Greek and Roman civilizations, Islamic culture, Christian communities, and many more.

This mix of cultures has resulted in a unique culinary tradition - based on fresh ingredients sourced from local markets.

From the Mediterranean coast to inland regions, the delicacies of paella, moussaka, tzatziki, lamb tagine, and seafood delights like calamari and octopus make delicious recipes and culinary combinations.

The influence of all the different cultures also means that the region's cuisine constantly evolves with fresh inspiration and new recipes.

Each recipe in this cookbook follows traditional flavors while incorporating a modernized approach to cooking—making it easy to stick with the Mediterranean diet while avoiding the fussiness of hard-to-make dishes.

From one-pot wonders like Savory Harissa Chickpea Stew over Creamy Millet and Eggplant to classic tomato-based creations like Spaghetti with Olives & Capers and Baked Ricotta & Spinach Pie with Feta Cheese—you'll be amazed at all that you can create in minutes!

Incorporating ingredients such as olive oil, herbs, spices, grains, and seafood into meals allows you to stay full and satisfied while staying within dietary guidelines.

Check out Nutiro.com or create a customized meal plan that makes it easy to plan what to eat for breakfast, lunch, dinner, or snacks, including keto, paleo, vegan, gluten-free, and vegetarian options.

What Foods Are in the Mediterranean Diet?

The Mediterranean diet is known for its rich variety of foods, flavors, and textures. As long as half the plate contains vegetables and grains, and meat is more of an afterthought or side dish to accompany the rest of the meal, the Mediterranean diet's basic principles are followed.

In order to get started with the Mediterranean diet, we have compiled a shopping list in the next section that will be a great guide on what foods to buy.

Planning for the Mediterranean Diet

It is easy making dishes Mediterranean-friendly. When concentrating on macronutrients, the Mediterranean diet is generally 50% carbohydrates, 15% protein, and 35% fat (Moore, 2020).

> The Mediterranean diet is adaptable and offers the freedom to customize macronutrient intake according to individual needs and preferences.

After preparing a Mediterranean meal, fill half the plate with vegetables, a quarter with grains, and the last quarter with protein—of which 10% should be healthy fats (Moore, 2020).

Meal prep is vital to any diet, as it prevents you from eating the same thing repeatedly, getting bored, or running into nutrient deficiencies. Meal prep is more than just thinking of what to eat next; it is about planning all meals and snacks several days in advance. Select several recipes, write down the quantities of ingredients needed, and then go shopping.

Preparing several meals early on a down day or weekend is an excellent tip for meal planning and preparation. This can save time and make it easier to stick to healthy eating habits throughout the week.

Meal planning is essential because it helps ensure that healthy and nutritious meals are readily available, ultimately leading to better health outcomes. Not everyone is capable or has the time to prepare a week's worth of food.

Start with some snacks and a few meals, and build it up to always have one day set aside to prepare your meals for the week. Preparing meals ahead of time can also help to reduce stress and make it easier to maintain a healthy diet, even on busy or tiring days.

Meats, vegetables, and grains can all be bulk bought and cooked ahead of time. These can then be portioned and used in a meal or frozen for later use. While most grains must be boiled, meat and vegetables can be grilled, air fried, or even roasted.

It isn't just full meals you should consider preparing ahead of time. Consider making fresh hummus to go with your precut vegetables. Even recipes, such as overnight oats, are a great way to ensure breakfast awaits you.

Lastly, don't be afraid to experiment with different types of recipes and foods to find those which you not only enjoy but can be stored for later use. There is no point in making a dish that will only last one day in the fridge if you are not planning on eating it immediately. Find recipes that suit not only your diet but also your taste.

Mediterranean Diet Shopping List

One of the hardest things to do when changing your diet is knowing what to buy and eat. While this is not a comprehensive list of what is eaten on the Mediterranean diet, this handy shopping list will guide you the next time you take a trip to your grocery store.

Food Types		Examples
Dairy	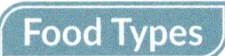	Greek yogurt (unsweetened), labneh, cheese (chevre, parmesan, ricotta, brie, halloumi, pecorino, manchego, feta, corvo), milk or milk alternatives (unsweetened soy, oats, pea, or almond milk).
Eggs		Eggs from chicken, duck, and quail.
Fats		Extra virgin olive oil (EVOO), ghee (clarified butter), avocado oil, and grapeseed oil.
Fruits		Grapes, pomegranates, apples, apricots, dates, figs, plums, apples, avocado, peaches, all berries, cherries, nectarines, oranges, grapefruit, lemons, tangerines, clementines, melons, bananas, olives, pears, and tomatoes.
Grains		Barley, oats, freekeh, bulgar, millet, rye, quinoa, couscous, buckwheat, and different kinds of rice (black, brown, wild, and others).
Legumes		Peanuts, chickpeas (can be used to make hummus), peas, lentils, and beans (cannellini, pinto, black, and others).
Meat	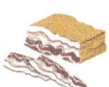	Lean pork, poultry, beef, lamb and mutton, duck, and guinea fowl.

Herbs		Mint, basil, bay leaves, parsley, oregano, cilantro, coriander, thyme, and marjoram. » Za'atar is a classic herb mixture often found in Mediterranean food. You can purchase it as is or find a recipe to make it. It contains thyme, marjoram, oregano, salt, sumac, and toasted sesame seeds.
Spices		Turmeric, allspice, cloves, black pepper, nutmeg, paprika, and saffron.
Seafood		Sardines, cod, salmon, yellowtail, mackerel, tilapia, sea bass, tuna, flounder, eel, shrimp, crab, lobster, abalone, cockles, mussels, oysters, whelks, clams, squid, and octopus.
Seeds and Nuts		Almonds, hazelnuts, pistachios, cashews, walnuts, chia, sunflower, pine nuts, pumpkin, sesame seeds, and flax.
Vegetables		Spinach, lettuce, radishes, potatoes, chicory, eggplant, okra, artichokes, Brussels sprouts, turnips, arugula, kale, peppers (all types), broccoli, dandelion greens, celeriac, onions (all types), tomatoes, celery, rutabaga, pumpkin, garlic, leeks, sweet potatoes, shallots, squashes (zucchini), collard greens, eggplant, beets, mushrooms, beans, mustard greens, cucumber, peas, carrots, garlic, and cabbage.

Now that you know what to buy, it's time to put the ingredients to work and make tasty Mediterranean meals.

Recipe Layout

Following a wholesome diet has never tasted so good! If you're longing for an indulgent and delicious diet that doesn't sacrifice flavor for a good lifestyle, then you'll enjoy the recipes contained in this book—from delicious appetizers to scrumptious desserts, you will find something to satisfy your cravings.

So, dive into the next chapter to experience the various recipes to give you a taste of what it's like to be within the Mediterranean region.

The book has sections for different recipes, including dinner, lunch, breakfast, and even snacks! Because of the adaptability of the Mediterranean diet, there are even chapters dedicated to diets such as keto, paleo, gluten-free, vegan, and vegetarian. Feel free to use any of the recipes, regardless of which sections they appear in.

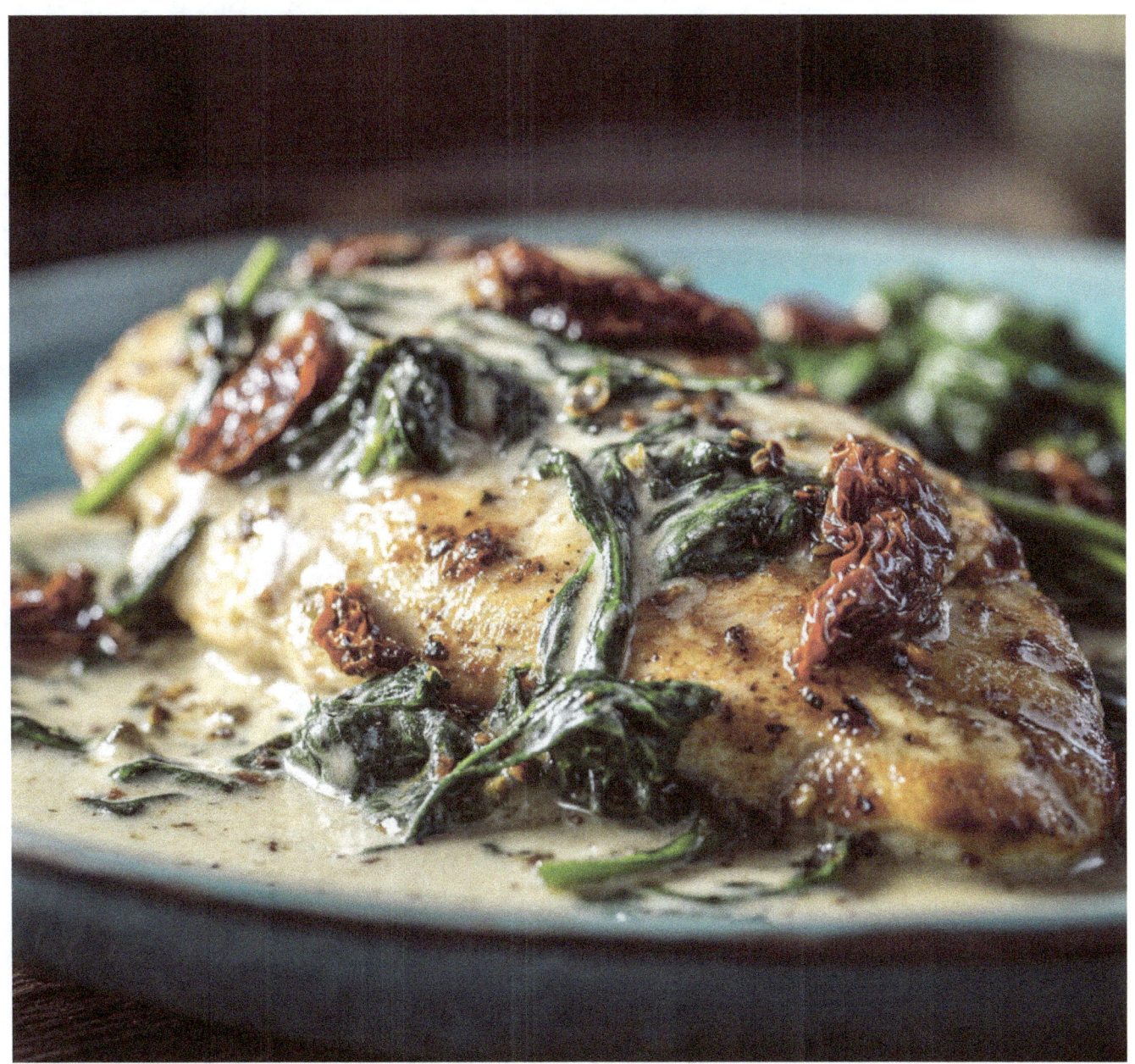

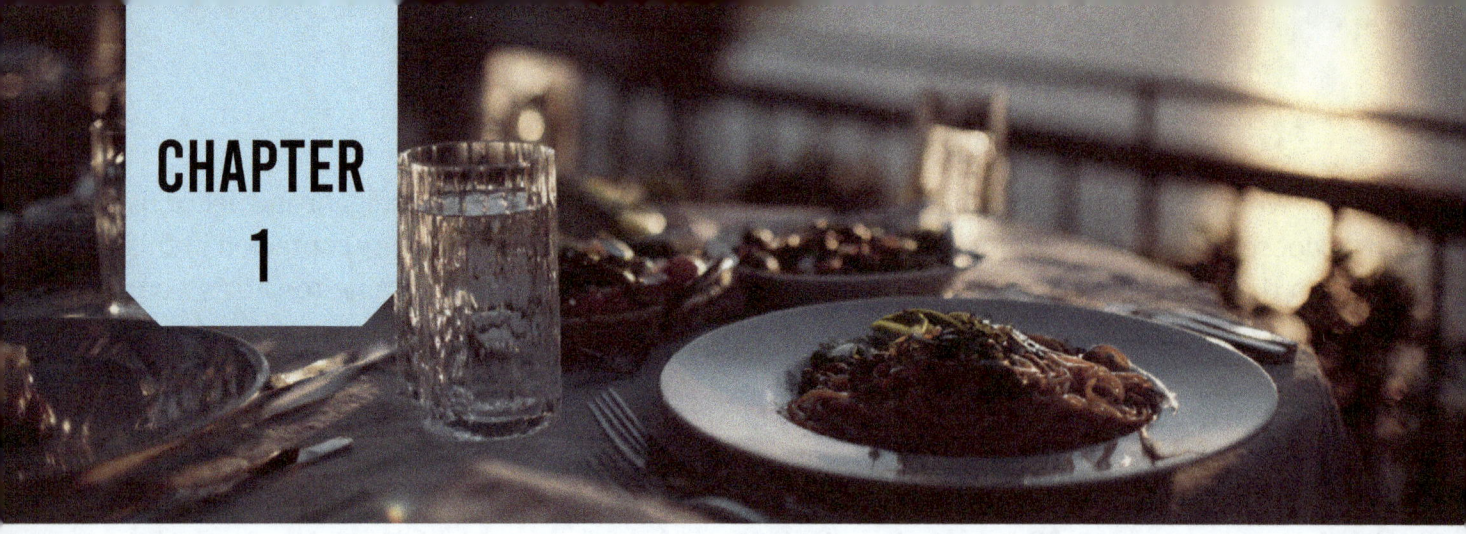

CHAPTER 1

Dinner MEDITERRANEAN Style

Enjoying a Mediterranean dinner is like taking a mini vacation to the Mediterranean Sea. From savory appetizers to succulent meats and fresh vegetables, you can experience all the flavors of the Mediterranean in one meal. The warm spices and herbs used provide an aromatic and flavorful backdrop that tantalizes your senses.

There is something special about sitting down to a meal with friends or family that features classic Mediterranean dishes that pack its own unique taste and texture, making it an unforgettable experience. Add some freshly baked flatbreads to dip in olive oil or tzatziki sauce for a truly authentic experience!

Smoked Salmon and Feta Fritters
(Gluten-Free + Keto-Friendly)

Not in the mood for a large dinner? Try a few salmon and feta fritters. The delicate taste of the salmon is elevated by the boldness of the feta, while the crispness of the mint leaves provides a refreshing balance. The fritters are enjoyable, hot or cold; they can last a few days in the fridge but longer in the freezer.

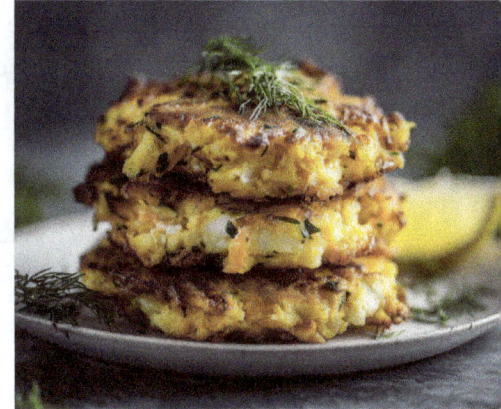

TIME: 37 MIN	SERVINGS: 4	PREP: 12 MIN	COOK: 25 MIN
CALORIES: 308 KCAL	CARBS: 38.5 G	FAT: 10.2 G	PROTEIN: 16.4 G

INGREDIENTS

- ½ cup cottage cheese
- ½ cup yogurt
- 1.8 oz feta cheese, crumbled
- 1 cup green salad
- 1 cup breadcrumbs, gluten-free
- 1 tbsp fresh mint, chopped finely
- 1 large egg, lightly beaten
- 2.6 oz smoked salmon, divided into 4 portions
- ¾ cup fresh corn kernels
- 1 medium zucchini, grated
- 1 lemon, quartered
- 1 pinch of ground black pepper

DIRECTIONS

1. Preheat the oven to 400° F.
2. Prepare an oven tray with baking paper and set it aside.
3. In a large bowl, add the pepper, mint, cheese, breadcrumbs, corn, egg, and zucchini before mixing.
4. Divide the contents into 8 portions for the fritters, then place them in the prepared tray.
5. Add the tray to the oven and bake until golden brown, roughly 25 minutes.
6. Once fully cooked, divide the fritters before serving them with yogurt, smoked salmon, and salad, accompanied by lemon wedges.

Marinated Chicken and Beef Kabobs

(Gluten-Free + Keto-Friendly)

These succulent kebabs are not only a delicious Mediterranean dish, but they're also quick and easy to make. These kabobs are perfect for any meal, so enjoy them with a Greek cucumber salad to make a complete dinner.

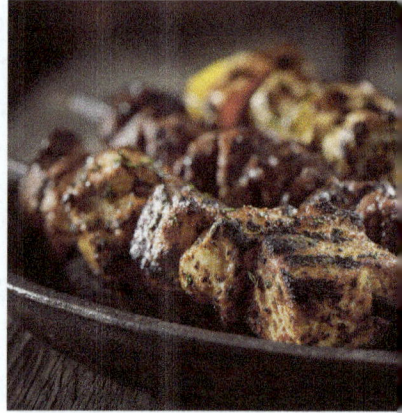

TIME: 22 MIN	SERVINGS: 4 (12 kabobs)	PREP: 10 MIN	COOK: 12 MIN
CALORIES: 249 KCAL	CARBS: 9.8 G	FAT: 11.1 G	PROTEIN: 27.1 G

INGREDIENTS

- 2 tbsp olive oil
- 12 wooden skewers
- 3 clove garlic, minced
- 6 oz beef sirloin strips, cut into 12 cubes
- 1 medium onion, cut into ¾ inch squares - create 12 cubes
- 2 tbsp lemon juice
- 1 medium red bell pepper, cut into 12 ¾ inch squares
- 6 oz chicken breast filet, cut into 12 cubes
- 1 tbsp fresh parsley
- 12 cherry tomatoes
- ½ tsp salt

DIRECTIONS

1. Heat the broiler up on high and place a rack 3 inches from the heat.
2. In a small bowl, mix the olive oil, salt, garlic, parsley, and lemon juice.
3. Divide between 2 bowls, 1 will be used for the raw meat, and the other for cooking and serving.
4. In a large bowl, combine the pepper, onions, chicken, beef, and tomatoes in a large bowl before pouring in the marinade. Mix until everything is well combined, and then allow the mixture to chill for 5 minutes.
5. After this, thread a cube of chicken, beef, onion, pepper, and tomato per skewer. Discard the leftover used marinade.
6. Place the skewers in the baking tray in the oven. Grill the kabobs for 3 minutes on each side while adding the fresh marinade until the meat is fully cooked.
7. Divide the skewers between 4 plates and drizzle the remaining marinade over the kebobs before serving.

Greek Moussaka

A traditional Greek dish featuring layers of eggplant, spiced ground meat, and creamy béchamel sauce. This hearty meal is perfect for a comforting dinner.

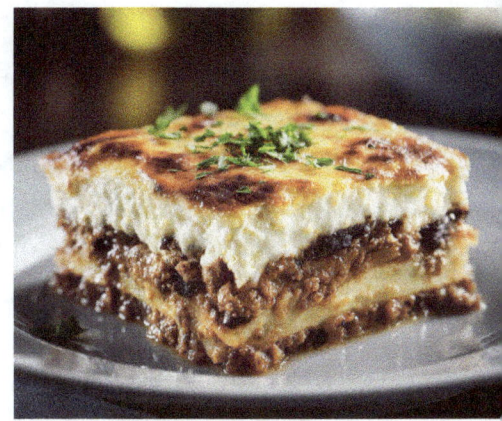

TIME: 1 H 30 MIN	SERVINGS: 6	PREP: 30 MIN	COOK: 1 H
CALORIES: 390 KCAL	CARBS: 20.5 G	FAT: 22.7 G	PROTEIN: 27.3 G

INGREDIENTS

Eggplant Layer Ingredients:
- 3 large eggplants, sliced into ¼-inch rounds
- 1 tsp salt
- 3 tbsp olive oil
- Meat Sauce Ingredients:
- 1 lb ground lamb or beef
- 1 onion, finely chopped
- 2 cloves garlic, minced
- 1 (14 oz) can crushed tomatoes
- 1 tsp cinnamon
- ½ tsp allspice
- 2 tbsp tomato paste
- ½ tsp salt
- ¼ tsp black pepper

Béchamel Sauce Ingredients:
- 2 cups milk (or unsweetened almond milk for Paleo-friendly)
- 2 tbsp ghee or butter
- 2 tbsp arrowroot flour or all-purpose flour
- ¼ tsp nutmeg
- ¼ tsp salt
- 1 large egg, lightly beaten

Topping Ingredients:
- ½ cup grated parmesan cheese (optional)

DIRECTIONS

1. Sprinkle the eggplant slices with salt and let them sit for 20 minutes to draw out moisture. Pat dry with paper towels.
2. Preheat the oven to 400°F. Arrange the slices on a baking sheet, brush with olive oil, and roast for 20 minutes, flipping halfway.
3. Heat olive oil in a skillet over medium heat. Add the onion and garlic, cooking until softened.
4. Add the ground meat, breaking it apart as it brown
5. Stir in the crushed tomatoes, tomato paste, cinnamon, allspice, salt, and pepper. Simmer for 20 minutes until thickened.
6. Prepare the Béchamel Sauce:

7. Heat ghee or butter in a saucepan over medium heat. Whisk in the arrowroot flour until smooth.
8. Gradually add the milk, whisking constantly, until the sauce thickens. Remove from heat and stir in nutmeg and salt.
9. Allow to cool slightly, then whisk in the beaten egg.
10. Assemble & Bake:
11. Reduce the oven temperature to 375°F.
12. In a greased baking dish, layer half the roasted eggplant slices, followed by the meat sauce. Repeat with the remaining eggplant slices.
13. Pour the béchamel sauce over the top and spread evenly. Sprinkle with parmesan cheese if desired.
14. Bake for 30-35 minutes, or until the top is golden and bubbling.
15. Allow the Moussaka to rest for 10 minutes before slicing. Serve warm and enjoy!

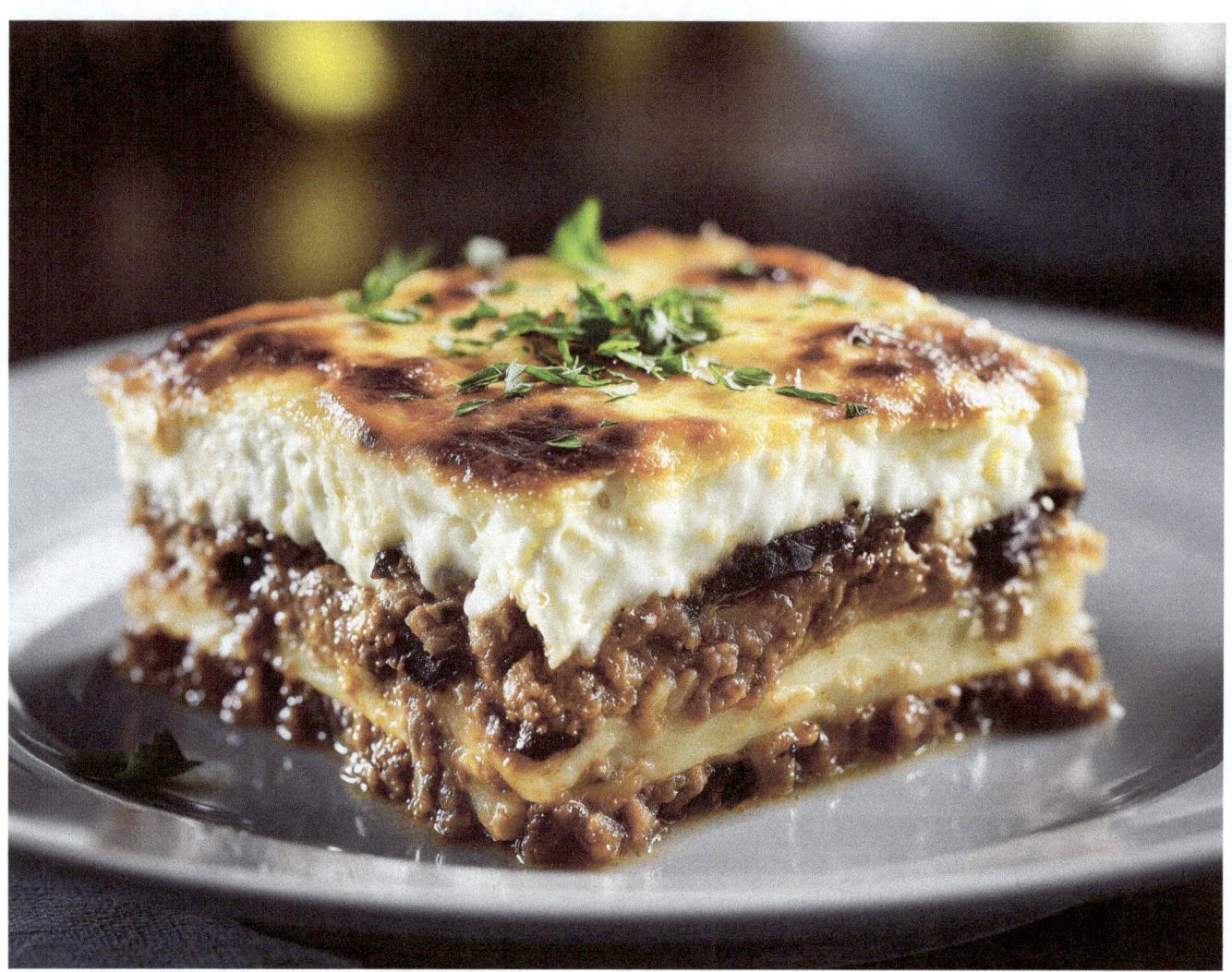

Spanish Paella

A classic Spanish dish featuring saffron-infused rice, seafood, and vibrant vegetables for a hearty and flavorful meal.

TIME: 1 H	SERVINGS: 6	PREP: 20 MIN	COOK: 40 MIN
CALORIES: 375 KCAL	CARBS: 42.7 G	FAT: 9.4 G	PROTEIN: 28.6 G

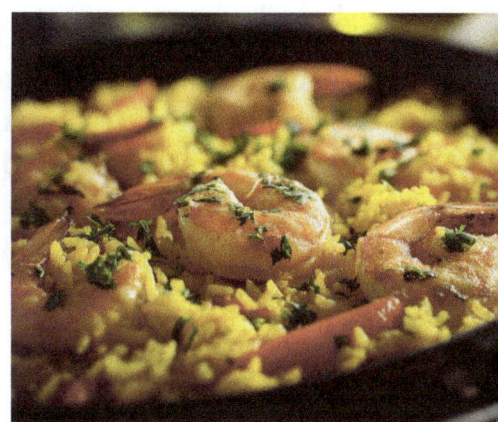

INGREDIENTS

- 2 tbsp olive oil
- 1 medium onion, finely chopped
- 3 cloves garlic, minced
- 1 red bell pepper, sliced
- 1 yellow bell pepper, sliced
- 2 medium tomatoes, grated (or 1 cup crushed tomatoes)
- 1½ cups short-grain rice (like Bomba or Arborio)
- ½ tsp salt
- ¼ tsp black pepper
- 1 tsp smoked paprika
- ½ tsp saffron threads (soaked in 2 tbsp warm water)
- 4 cups chicken or seafood broth
- ½ lb shrimp, peeled and deveined
- ½ lb mussels, cleaned
- ½ lb clams, cleaned
- 1 cup frozen peas, thawed
- Lemon wedges, for garnish

DIRECTIONS

1. Heat olive oil in a large, deep skillet or paella pan over medium heat.
2. Sauté the onion and garlic until soft, about 2-3 minutes.
3. Add the bell peppers and cook for 5 minutes until tender.
4. Stir in the grated tomatoes, smoked paprika, and saffron with its soaking water. Cook for 3-4 minutes until the mixture thickens slightly.
5. Stir the rice into the pan, coating it in the tomato mixture. Cook for 1-2 minutes to toast the rice lightly.
6. Add the broth, salt, and pepper. Stir once to combine, then spread the mixture evenly in the pan.
7. Reduce the heat to medium-low and simmer without stirring for 15-20 minutes, or until the rice is almost cooked and most of the liquid is absorbed.
8. Nestle the shrimp, mussels, and clams into the rice, and scatter the peas on top.
9. Cover the pan with a lid or foil and cook for another 8-10 minutes, or until the seafood is cooked and the mussels and clams have opened.
10. Remove from heat and let the paella rest, covered, for 5 minutes. Garnish with lemon wedges and serve warm.

Sesame Chicken with Snap Peas and Peppers

Chicken doesn't need to be boring! With the addition of peppers and snap peas to this dish, this recipe produces a sweet and tangy dinner you may struggle to share. For extra flavor, be sure to roast the sesame seeds. It'll surely make the dish pop even more!

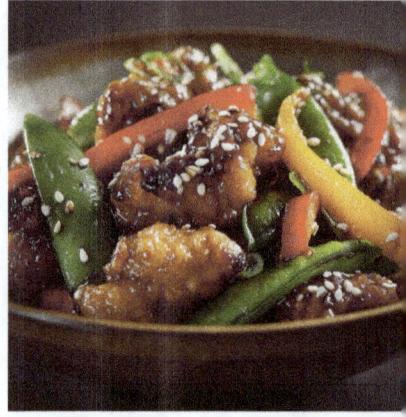

TIME: 25 MIN	SERVINGS: 4	PREP: 5 MIN	COOK: 20 MIN
CALORIES: 363 KCAL	CARBS: 27.8 G	FAT: 10.3 G	PROTEIN: 38.6 G

INGREDIENTS

- 2 cups brown rice, cooked
- 1 tbsp sesame seeds
- 1 red bell pepper, chopped
- 2 green onions sliced
- 1 tsp salt
- 1 lb chicken breast, cut into strips
- ¼ tsp ground ginger
- 1 green bell pepper, chopped
- 2 cups snap peas
- 1 ½ tsp honey
- 2 tbsp water

DIRECTIONS

1. Heat a skillet over medium-high and add sesame seeds. Toast the seeds until light brown then set aside.
2. Before adding the chicken strips, drizzle a bit of oil into the skillet. Cook at medium-high for 10 minutes or until done.
3. Once the chicken is cooked, add the bell peppers and peas, then stir fry for another 3 minutes. Ensure the vegetables remain crisp and tender.
4. In a clean bowl, pour in the water, salt, ginger, and honey, and mix until the honey is dissolved. Drizzle over the skillet mixture and cook for another 5 minutes at medium-high.
5. Split the rice between 4 bowls, add ¾ cup of the skillet contents, and then sprinkle with green onions and sesame seeds before serving.

Mediterranean Gnocchi
(Vegetarian-Friendly)

This Italian dish is vibrantly colorful and can easily be thrown together when purchasing grilled vegetables. Seek out colorful peppers, sweet onions, mild eggplant, and some tangy artichoke to grill at home to ensure your plate is as colorful and tasty as possible.

TIME: 40 MIN	SERVINGS: 2	PREP: 10 MIN	COOK: 30 MIN
CALORIES: 353 KCAL	CARBS: 68 G	FAT: 5 G	PROTEIN: 7 G

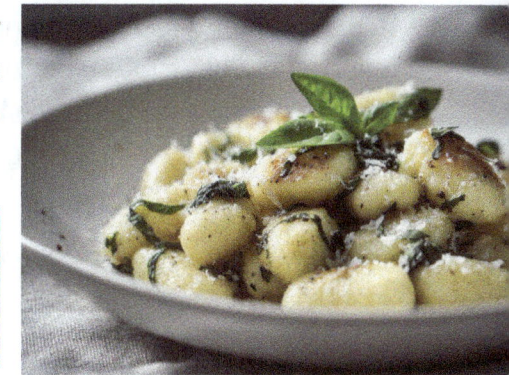

INGREDIENTS

FOR RED PESTO:
- 8 oz sun-dried tomatoes packed in oil, undrained
- 3 garlic cloves
- ½ cup fresh basil leaves, packed (slightly squashed into measuring tool
- 1 roasted red pepper, from a jar
- ½ cup parmesan cheese, freshly grated
- ¼ tsp salt
- ¼ cup fresh parsley leaves, packed (slightly squashed into measuring tool)
- ¼ tsp pepper
- olive oil, as needed

FOR GNOCCHI:
- 2 oz peppers, chopped
- 2 oz eggplant, chopped
- 1 oz artichokes, chopped
- 1 oz cherry tomatoes, halved
- 1 oz onions, sliced
- 14 oz gnocchi
- a handful of basil leaves
- 2 tbsp red pesto
- Sea salt for pasta water
- 1 tbsp parmesan, to serve

DIRECTIONS

FOR RED PESTO:
1. Add tomatoes, basil, garlic, roasted pepper, parsley, and parmesan to a food processor and blend until a thick paste develops.
2. Pour a teaspoon of olive oil at a time and continue to blend until the pesto is smooth.
3. Add the salt and pepper, season to taste.
4. Pesto will last 3 days in the fridge and 3 months in the freezer.

FOR GNOCCHI:
1. In a pot, add salted water and gnocchi, then cook until the pieces rise to the surface (or follow box instructions).
2. As the gnocchi cooks, add the vegetables to a tray with olive oil and grill for 20–25 minutes.
3. Decant (pour off) some of the cooking water and keep it while the rest of the pot is drained. Replace the gnocchi and the retained cooking water.
4. Add the pieces of chargrilled vegetables, basil leaves, and red pesto before stirring.
5. Serve with some parmesan.

Chicken, Vegetables, and Risoni Salad
(Gluten-Free)

Dressing up chicken for dinner has never been easier. Enjoy oven-roasted sweet potatoes, zucchini, onion, pepper, and asparagus, together with sliced chicken breast on risoni rice smothered in a tangy yogurt dressing to enjoy and even reheat throughout the week.

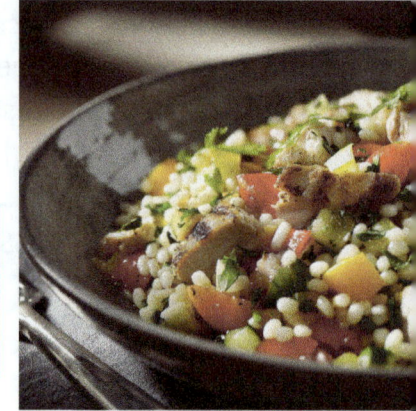

TIME: 45 MIN	SERVINGS: 4	PREP: 10 MIN + 10 MIN Cooling	COOK: 25 MIN
CALORIES: 366 KCAL	CARBS: 42.1 G	FAT: 8.5 G	PROTEIN: 27.4 G

INGREDIENTS

- 8.8 oz chicken breast, cut into inch-sized cubes or slices
- 1 cup gluten-free risoni pasta, cooked in salt water until al dente
- 7 oz sweet potato, cut into inch cubes
- 1 red onion, cut into thin wedges
- 1 sweet red pepper, cut into inch rounds
- 1 zucchini, cut into inch rounds
- ½ cup asparagus, cut into two-inch lengths
- 1 cup yogurt
- ½ tsp salt
- 1 tsp ground paprika
- 1 pinch of ground black pepper
- 3 clove garlic, crushed
- 2 tsp olive oil
- ½ cup fresh parsley chopped
- 2 tsp red wine vinegar

DIRECTIONS

1. While preheating the oven to 350° F, place baking paper on an oven tray.
2. In a large bowl, add the vegetables, chicken, oil, salt paprika, and garlic before mixing well.
3. Be sure the mixture is laid in a single layer on the tray and bake for 25 minutes. Ensure the chicken is fully cooked.
4. Remove from the oven and allow the tray to sit undisturbed for 10 minutes.
5. In a smaller bowl, mix the vinegar and yogurt.
6. Remove the chicken from the tray and slice thinly before adding it to a large bowl with the roasted vegetables, the risoni, parsley, and half of the dressing. Add the pepper to taste.
7. Toss mixture to coat well and serve hot or cold.

Mediterranean and Basil Pasta
(Vegetarian-Friendly)

The Mediterranean and basil pasta is a win-win recipe, regardless of being served hot or cold. Enjoy delicious pasta topped with sweet red peppers, mildly spicy chilies, and sunkissed tomatoes. Don't forget to add the fresh basil at the end to experience its savory-sweet aroma.

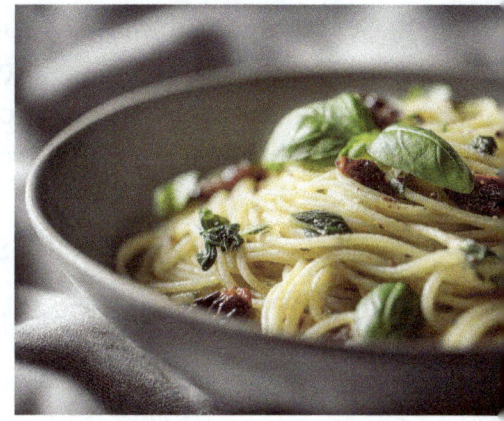

TIME: 35 MIN	SERVINGS: 4	PREP: 5 MIN	COOK: 30 MIN
CALORIES: 452 KCAL	CARBS: 86 G	FAT: 8 G	PROTEIN: 14 G

INGREDIENTS

- 2 red peppers, seeded and cut coarsely
- 12 oz dried pasta
- 2 red onions, cut into wedges
- 2.2 lb small ripe tomatoes, quartered
- 2 mild red chilies, seeded and diced
- 1 tsp honey
- 3 garlic cloves, coarsely chopped
- ¼ tsp salt
- ¼ tsp pepper
- 2 tbsp olive oil, to serve
- 2 tbsp grated parmesan, to serve
- fresh basil leaves, to serve

DIRECTIONS

1. Preheat the oven to 400 °F.
2. In an oven tray, add the red peppers, garlic, chilies, and onions, and drizzle with oil, salt, pepper, and honey.
3. Grill mixed vegetables for 15 minutes before adding tomatoes and roasting for another 15 minutes.
4. As the vegetables are roasting, cook the pasta until al dente before draining.
5. In a large bowl, add the roasted vegetables and pour in the pasta before tossing lightly.
6. To finish, gently tear the basil leaves and scatter them and add a sprinkle of parmesan over the mixture.

All-In-One Fish Supper
(Paleo-Friendly + Gluten-Free)

Get transported with these delicious and unforgettable Mediterranean flavors. The nutty tang of artichoke hearts is enhanced by the sprinkle of the saltiness of the prosciutto, and the two together help to strengthen the delicate flavor of the fish.

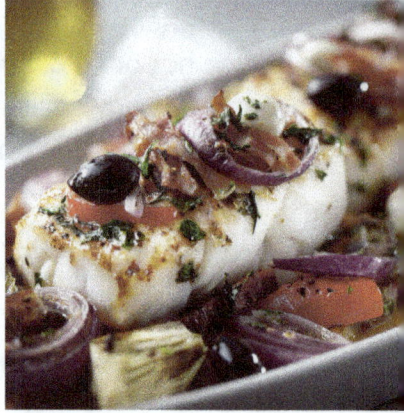

TIME: 42 MIN	SERVINGS: 2	PREP: 15 MIN	COOK: 27 MIN
CALORIES: 521 KCAL	CARBS: 26 G	FAT: 28 G	PROTEIN: 40 G

INGREDIENTS

- 2 slices prosciutto, cut in half
- ½ tsp chili paste or powder
- 3 tbsp olive oil
- 10 oz jar artichoke hearts, drained
- 2 red peppers, sliced thinly
- 2 garlic cloves, sliced thinly
- handful black olives
- 2 red onions, sliced thinly
- 4 fish filets, bass or bream
- splash of white wine

DIRECTIONS

1. In a large pan, add some oil and prosciutto pieces, and then cook until crispy before setting aside.
2. Add the garlic, peppers, and onions to the same pan and add the remaining oil before cooking for another 10 minutes, stirring now and again, until everything is softened.
3. Pour in the wine, artichoke hearts, chili, and olives, and cook 1–2 minutes longer.
4. Lay the filets over the vegetables and cover the pan, then cook for another 5–6 minutes.
5. Once the fish are cooked through, scatter the prosciutto over the top and serve with some crusty gluten-free bread.

Saffron Lamb Tagine
(Gluten-Free)

This saffron lamb tagine may not be cooked in a classic Moroccan tagine, but it'll be well worth it. Not only is it mouthwatering, but it's flavorful, colorful, and fragrant. You can even cook this hearty meal in a pot on the stove!

TIME: 1 Hr 55 MIN	SERVINGS: 4	PREP: 40 MIN	COOK: 1 Hr 15 MIN
CALORIES: 606 KCAL	CARBS: 73.8 G	FAT: 13.1 G	PROTEIN: 46.4 G

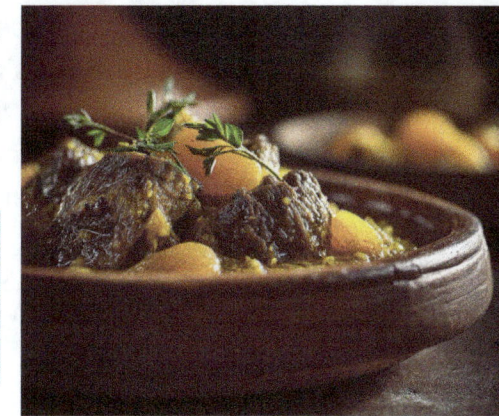

INGREDIENTS

- 1 ½ cups yogurt
- 14.1 oz leg of lamb, cut into inch pieces
- 14.1 oz chickpeas, drained and rinsed
- 4.4 oz quinoa
- 14 fluid oz chicken broth
- ½ tsp sea salt
- 1 tsp ground turmeric
- 2 tsp ground coriander
- 2 tsp ground cumin
- 2 tsp ground ginger
- 2 tsp ground cinnamon
- 2 medium red onions, julienned (cut into fine strips)
- 3 oz dates, cut lengthwise
- 2 clove garlic, crushed
- 1 tsp olive oil
- ¾ cup baby carrots, cut in half lengthwise
- 1 small pinch of saffron
- 2 tsp sesame seeds, toasted
- 2 tbsp coriander leaves, garnish

DIRECTIONS

1. In a flat container, add ½ cup of yogurt and mix in the spices and garlic. Add the lamb and mix until coated. Place the container in the fridge and marinate for 30 minutes.
2. Bring chicken broth to a boil, and turn off to bloom saffron in broth for 15 minutes.
3. Once the meat is marinated, add a pan to medium heat and heat the oil before adding ¾ of the cut onions. Cook until tender, 5 minutes. The remaining uncooked onion will be served with the meal.
4. Remove the lamb from the fridge and cook with onion over medium heat for about 5 minutes.
5. Pour in the stock, chickpeas, and dates before bringing the mixture to a boil, and then lower it to a simmer. Place the lid onto the pot and simmer for 30 minutes.
6. Cut baby carrots in half and add to pot. Place the lid onto the pot and simmer for another 30 minutes until the meat is tender (about an hour total cook time).
7. Once the meat has reached its desired level of tenderness, remove the lid and let the mixture simmer for an additional 5 minutes. This will allow the sauce to reduce, enhancing its flavors and texture.
8. Serve the succulent lamb with onion slices, the remaining yogurt, and a dash of coriander. Once plated, lightly sprinkle sesame seeds over the lamb tagine, add a side of quinoa, sprinkle a light dusting of coriander powder; garnish with coriander leaves to complete this wholesome dish.

Rosemary Grilled Lamb Chops
(Gluten-Free)

Grilled lamb chops make a perfect light dinner, and with an apple and mint sauce, this recipe gives you a unique blend of tastes. Enjoy these chops with a large plate of Greek salad (from the Stuffed Avocados recipe) or cooked mixed vegetables such as the steamed collard greens from the Mediterranean Marinated Tenderloin recipe.

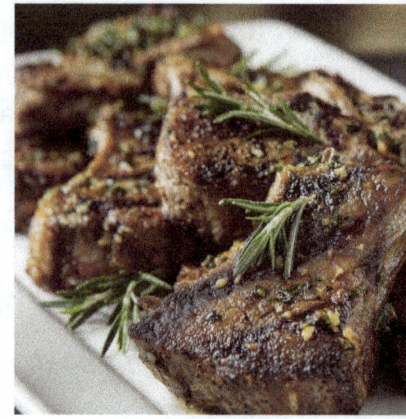

TIME: 50 MIN	SERVINGS: 8 (8 chops)	PREP: 40 MIN	COOK: 10 MIN
CALORIES: 386 KCAL	CARBS: 4 G	FAT: 37 G	PROTEIN: 9 G

INGREDIENTS

FOR MINT APPLE SAUCE:
- 3 sprigs of flat-leaf parsley, only leaves
- 1 tbsp lemon juice
- 1 Granny Smith apple, cored and sliced
- ⅓ cup olive oil
- ½ cup mint leaves, packed (slightly squashed into measuring tool)

FOR LAMB CHOPS:
- 1 rack of lamb, cut into individual chops
- ¼ cup olive oil
- 3 cloves garlic, minced
- ½ tsp salt
- 2 tsp fresh rosemary, finely chopped
- ¼ tsp pepper

DIRECTIONS

1. Add all the ingredients for the mint apple sauce to a food processor and pulse for a few minutes until well combined.
2. Scrape out the sauce and place it in a glass jar before adding it to the fridge until ready to use.
3. In a baking dish, add the garlic, rosemary, and olive oil before mixing well.
4. Add the chops to the baking dish, coat both sides with the mixture, then place in the fridge to marinate for 30 minutes.
5. Before grilling the chops, preheat your grill to medium-high heat. Cook each side for approximately 3-5 minutes or until the desired doneness. Once done, let the chops rest for a few minutes to allow the juices to settle before serving.
6. Spoon the remaining lamb jus marinade from the backing dish over the meat, and add the mint apple sauce to the side; serve immediately.

Spanish Meatball and Bean Stew
(Gluten-Free)

Warm, hearty, and bursting with Spanish flavors, this stew combines tender beef meatballs, buttery beans, and a rich tomato base seasoned with sweet smoked paprika and honey. Packed with vibrant red onion, colorful peppers, and fresh parsley, it's a wholesome meal perfect for chilly evenings. Pair it with gluten-free bread for a comforting and satisfying dish that's naturally gluten-free.

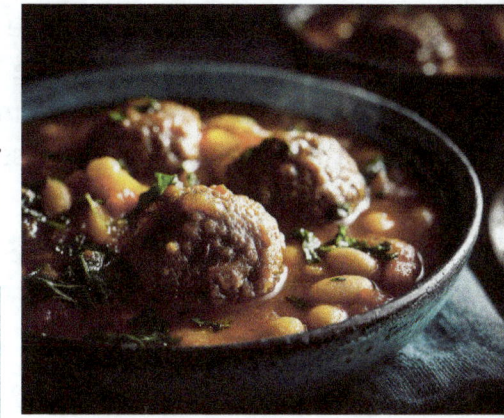

TIME: 25 MIN	SERVINGS: 3	PREP: 15 MIN	COOK: 35 MIN
CALORIES: 451 KCAL	CARBS: 38.9 G	FAT: 13.5 G	PROTEIN: 43.5 G

INGREDIENTS

- 12.3 oz ground lean beef
- 14 oz can butter beans, drained
- 2 tsp olive oil
- 2 (14 oz) cans chopped tomatoes
- 1 large red onion, chopped
- small bunch parsley, chopped
- 2 peppers, any color and sliced
- 1 tbsp sweet smoked paprika
- 2 tsp honey
- 3 garlic cloves, crushed
- gluten-free bread, to serve (optional)
- ¼ tsp salt
- ¼ tsp pepper

DIRECTIONS

1. Season the meat with a ¼ teaspoon of salt and pepper, and work the seasoning through with your hands before shaping it into small balls.
2. Add the meatballs and the oil to a large pan and cook until golden brown, roughly 5 minutes.
3. Move the meatballs to 1 side of the pan before adding the onions and peppers. Cook for 5 minutes until soft.
4. Add the garlic and paprika before stirring everything together for a minute.
5. Pour in the tomatoes before covering the pan and allowing the mixture to simmer for 10 minutes.
6. After simmering, add the honey, beans, and any seasoning if needed, and allow the contents to simmer without a lid for 10 minutes.
7. But before serving, stir in the parsley, and serve with some crusty bread.

Fish and Lemony Potatoes
(Gluten-Free)

While pollack tends to have a delicate and mild flavor, the kalamata olives help to highlight the unique flavor without overpowering it. Add this with the unique lemony baby potatoes, and you have a dish that will satisfy even the fussiest of eaters at dinnertime.

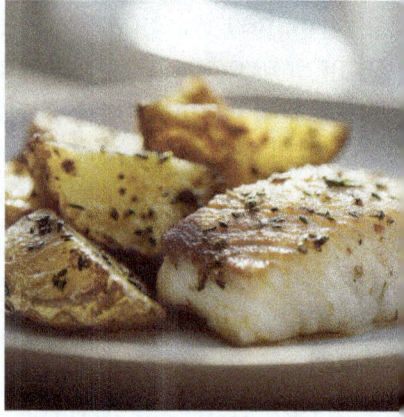

TIME: 30 MIN	SERVINGS: 2	PREP: 10 MIN	COOK: 20 MIN
CALORIES: 320 KCAL	CARBS: 23 G	FAT: 17 G	PROTEIN: 20.9 G

INGREDIENTS

- 10.5 oz baby potatoes
- 3.5 oz green beans
- 2 chunky pollock filets or white fish
- small handful black kalamata olives
- 2 tbsp olive oil
- zest and juice 1 lemon
- few tarragon sprigs, leaves only
- ¼ tsp salt
- ¼ tsp pepper

DIRECTIONS

1. Heat the oven to 400 °F.
2. Boil the potatoes in a pot of water for 10–12 minutes or until you can pierce them with a fork.
3. Add the beans to the potatoes and cook for 2–3 minutes before draining.
4. Cut the potatoes in half and place them in a large baking dish with the beans, lemon juice, lemon zest, and olives. Season with half of the salt and pepper.
5. Season the fish and then place the fish and then place remaining salt and pepper, season the fish, and then place it on top of the potato mixture.
6. Bake until the fish is fully cooked (about 10–12 minutes).
7. Remove the baking dish and add a splash of lemon juice before scattering the tarragon leaves over the top.
8. Serve while hot.

Mediterranean Marinated Tenderloin
(Gluten-Free)

While the sweet, spicy, and savory tang is reminiscent of south Asia, it contains many ingredients welcomed in the Mediterranean lifestyle. The fiery nature of fresh ginger is an excellent complement to pork, while the nutty undertones of the sesame oil remain hidden until you take your first bite. Enjoy on a bed of steamed collard greens or kale.

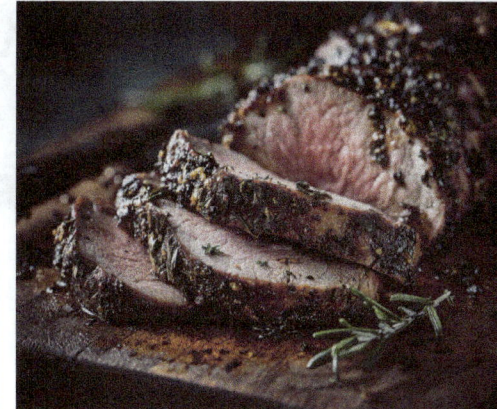

TIME: 1 Hr 20 MIN	SERVINGS: 4	PREP: 20 MIN	COOK: 60 MIN
CALORIES: 431 KCAL	CARBS: 3.6 G	FAT: 17.4 G	PROTEIN: 61.9 G

INGREDIENTS

FOR PORK:
- 2 lbs pork tenderloin
- 1 clove garlic
- ½ tbsp honey
- 2 tbsp fresh ginger, minced
- 1 tbsp soy sauce, gluten-free
- 1 tbsp fish sauce
- 1 tbsp sesame oil (optional)

FOR STEAMED COLLARD GREENS:
- 4 tsp virgin olive oil
- 40 whole leaves of collard greens, washed
- ¼ tsp salt
- 2 tbsp freshly grated Parmesan cheese (optional)

DIRECTIONS

1. Preheat the oven broiler to high and place a rack within 3 inches of the element.
2. Trim visible fat from the tenderloin and place the meat in a large oven dish.
3. In a small bowl, whisk together the garlic, ginger, honey, sesame oil, soy sauce, and fish sauce.
4. Pour ⅓ of the mixture over the tenderloin and place it in the oven.
5. Cook the pork, ensuring it reaches an internal temperature of 160°F. Baste the meat with a tablespoon of the marinade every 5 minutes. This process may take up to 50 minutes, so continue basting regularly for maximum flavor and tenderness.
6. While the meat is cooking, prepare the collard greens by trimming the hard stems.
7. Add the collard greens to a large saucepan with a cup of cold water. Bring to a boil, add salt, cover, and blanch for 5–10 minutes until tender and wilted.
8. Drain the greens, pat dry, and toss with Parmesan.
9. Once the tenderloin is fully cooked, remove it from the oven and let it rest for 5 minutes before slicing into 1-inch-thick pieces.
10. Serve 3 slices of tenderloin with the prepared steamed collard greens.

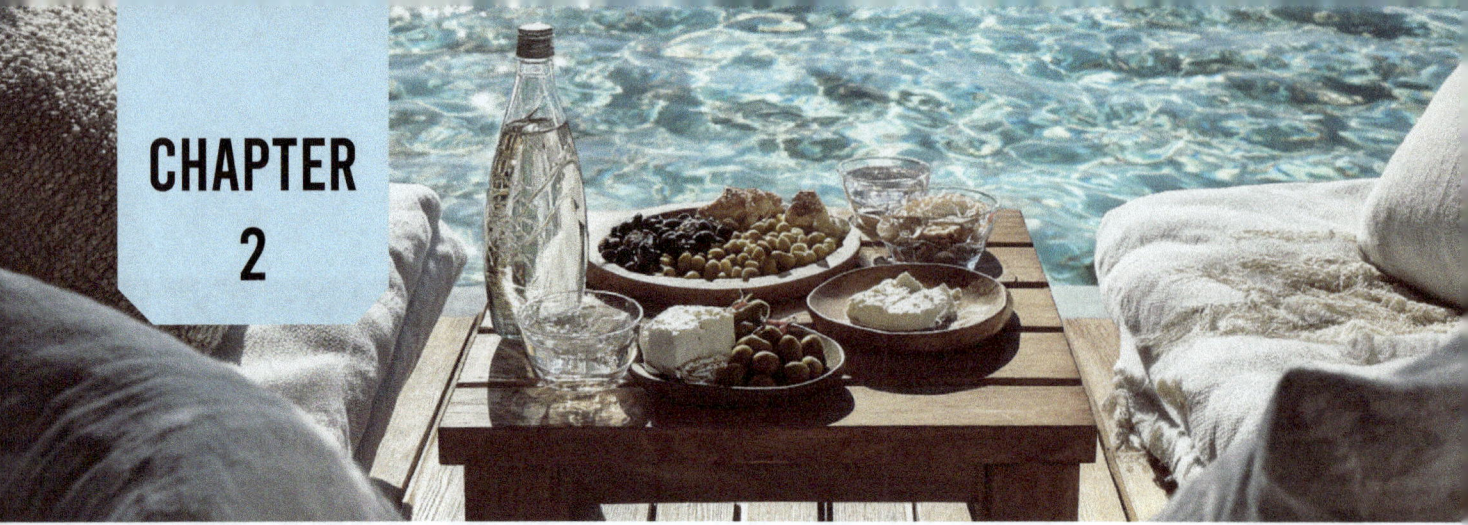

CHAPTER 2

Lunch MEDITERRANEAN Style

Enjoying a Mediterranean lunch is the perfect way to add some delightful flavors to your midday meal. Choose from a variety of spices such as paprika, oregano, and cumin to make your meal truly unique.

Opt for grilled chicken or fish paired with flavorful sides like char-grilled stuffed eggplant, savory harissa chickpea stew, or roasted vegetables with quinoa. Complete your meal with a sweet and fruity baklava for dessert or a refreshing zesty lemon sorbet.

Grilled Tuna with Spinach and Chickpeas
(Gluten-Free)

This nutrient-dense meal is satisfying and filling. By incorporating omega-3 fatty acids into this nutrient-dense meal, you're fulfilling your hunger and fueling your body with essential nutrients that have numerous health benefits.

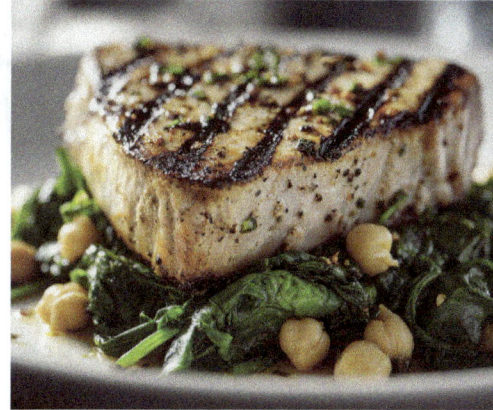

TIME: 18 MIN	SERVINGS: 4	PREP: 10 MIN	COOK: 8 MIN
CALORIES: 335 KCAL	CARBS: 29.7 G	FAT: 9.9 G	PROTEIN: 32.8 G

INGREDIENTS

- 2 tbsp lemon juice
- 15 oz chickpeas, drained and rinsed
- 1 medium tomato, cut into wedges
- 1 tbsp olive oil
- 1 tsp ground oregano
- 10 oz baby spinach, rinsed and dried
- ⅛ tsp ground black pepper
- 3 clove garlic, minced
- 1 tbsp lemon juice
- 12 oz tuna steak, quartered
- ⅛ tsp salt

DIRECTIONS

1. Preheat the oven broiler and place a rack within 3 inches of the heat.
2. In a bowl, pour the lemon juice, oil, and oregano. Allow the fish to marinate in the mixture for 5 minutes.
3. Add the remaining salad ingredients to a large bowl and refrigerate.
4. Remove the fish from the marinade and grill for 4 minutes per side or until they flake easily.
5. Serve the fish hot over a cup of the prepared salad.

Mediterranean Marinated Flank Steak
(Gluten-Free)

A grilled steak is one thing, but one marinated with the flavors of the Mediterranean is out of this world. The delicate balance of the herbs and red wine not only brings out the flavors of the meat but truly makes one believe that they're enjoying steak alongside the Mediterranean ocean. Serve alongside a tangy cucumber salad.

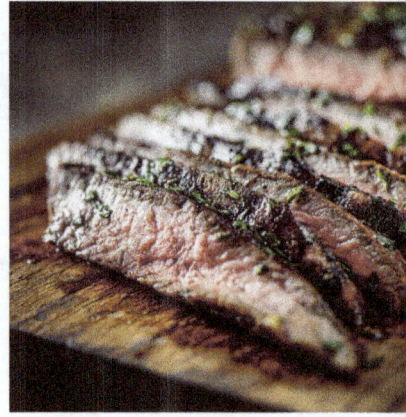

TIME: 46 MIN	SERVINGS: 4	PREP: 30 MIN	COOK: 16 MIN
CALORIES: 925 KCAL	CARBS: 1.9 G	FAT: 76.1 G	PROTEIN: 49.8 G

INGREDIENTS

FOR STEAK:
- 4 (10-12 oz) rib-eye steaks, cut to an inch thick
- 4 tsp salt

FOR MARINADE:
- ½ cup dry red wine
- 1 tsp dried thyme
- 1 tsp crushed red pepper flakes
- ¼ cup olive oil
- 2 tbsp fresh lemon juice
- 1 tsp dried marjoram
- 1 tsp garlic salt

DIRECTIONS

1. Add all the marinade ingredients to a large Ziplock bag, seal, and shake until well combined.
2. Add the steaks to the bag and squeeze all the air out before sealing again.
3. Turn the bag several times to distribute the marinade. Leave to marinate in the fridge for 30 minutes.
4. Remove the steaks from the bag and allow excess marinade to drip off before seasoning both sides with a teaspoon of salt.
5. In a nonstick pan place the steaks over high heat in a nonstick pan and cook for 6–8 minutes. Cook for less or more depending on how you prefer your steak's doneness.

Savory Harissa Chickpea Stew Over Creamy Millet

(Gluten-Free, Vegetarian-Friendly + Vegan-Friendly)

There's no need to eat meat with every meal with this delicious grain bowl full of vegetables to remind you of those Mediterranean winters. This comforting stew is perfectly seasoned to please even the pickiest of eaters.

TIME: 45 MIN	SERVINGS: 2	PREP: 10 MIN	COOK: 35 MIN
CALORIES: 600 KCAL	CARBS: 100 G	FAT: 15 G	PROTEIN: 20 G

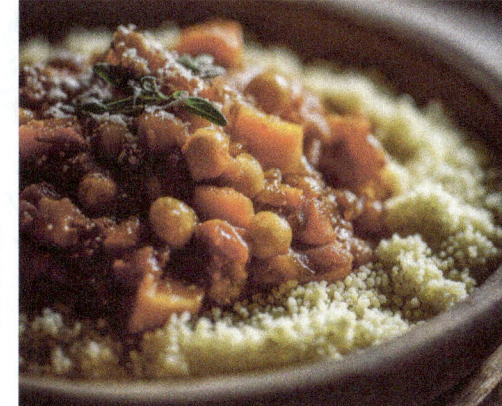

INGREDIENTS

- 1 large eggplant
- 1 cup millet
- 1 (14 oz) can purée tomatoes
- 2 tbsp harissa paste
- 2 tbsp olive oil, divided
- 1 (14 oz) can chickpeas, drained
- 3 garlic cloves, minced
- 1 onion, diced
- ¼ tsp pepper
- ¼ tsp salt
- 1 bunch cilantro, garnish

DIRECTIONS

1. In a medium saucepan, bring to boil the millet, 2 cups of water, and a pinch of salt. Lower the temperature to a simmer, cover the saucepan, and cook for 25 minutes. After, remove the cover, fluff the grain with a fork, and allow the millet to cool.
2. While the millet is cooking, add a tablespoon of oil to a deep skillet, then add the pepper, salt, and eggplant. Cook over medium heat for 10 minutes. Set aside.
3. In the same skillet, add another tablespoon of oil with the onions, and continue to cook for 8–10 minutes until soft before adding the garlic. Cook for another 2 minutes.
4. Lower the heat by adding the harissa, tomatoes, chickpeas, and eggplant. Allow the mixture to simmer for 10–15 minutes. Season to taste.
5. Scoop half the millet and top it with the hot stew. Sprinkle it with some cilantro and serve immediately.

Roasted Vegetable and Quinoa Bowl
(Gluten-Free + Vegetarian-Friendly)

This quinoa bowl is colorful, tasty, and has a beautiful and rich texture. The combination of ingredients creates a visually appealing dish, while the different textures add depth and interest to each bite. It's always a bonus when healthy food is also delicious, and this quinoa bowl sounds like it hits all the right notes.

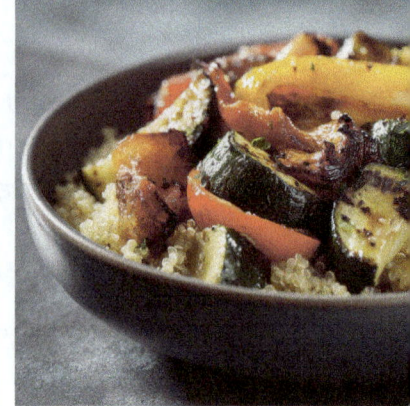

TIME: 50 MIN	SERVINGS: 4	PREP: 10 MIN	COOK: 40 MIN
CALORIES: 862 KCAL	CARBS: 96 G	FAT: 42 G	PROTEIN: 32 G

INGREDIENTS

- 1 large eggplant, cubed
- juice from ½ lemon
- 1 medium zucchini, cubed
- 1 garlic clove, minced
- 1 pint cherry tomatoes, sliced in half
- 1 cup of labneh or Greek yogurt
- a handful of romano beans
- ½ cup pesto
- olive oil
- 1 cup quinoa, rinsed
- handful of cilantro or parsley, roughly chopped
- ¼ tsp salt
- ¼ tsp pepper

DIRECTIONS

1. Preheat the oven to 400 °F.
2. Spread parchment paper on a large baking sheet and scatter the cherry tomatoes, beans, eggplant, and zucchini before drizzling the oil and seasoning with salt and pepper.
3. Roast the vegetable until tender (30–40 minutes).
4. While roasting the vegetables, add the quinoa to a saucepan with a pinch of salt and 2 cups of water. Bring the water up to a boil before lowering it to a simmer. Keep the quinoa simmering for 15 minutes in a covered saucepan.
5. After cooking, remove the lid, fluff the quinoa, and set it aside to cool before adding the pesto. Toss to coat the quinoa.
6. In a small bowl, add the labneh, lemon juice, herbs, and garlic in a small bowl, and mix.
7. Split the quinoa between 4 bowls, group the vegetables with their vibrant colors, and add a dollop of labneh to finish the presentation before serving.

Stuffed Eggplant

This stuffed eggplant recipe is a delicious and healthy dish that's perfect for dinner parties or a weeknight meal. Bursting with flavor and texture, the eggplants are halved and roasted until tender, then filled with a flavorful mixture of sautéed vegetables, then baked until golden brown.

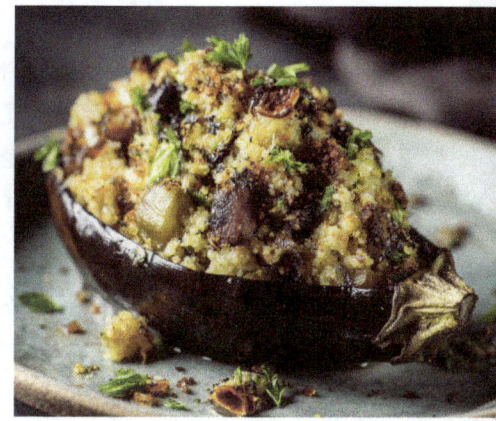

TIME: 45 MIN	SERVINGS: 4	PREP: 15 MIN	COOK: 30 MIN
CALORIES: 339 KCAL	CARBS: 46 G	FAT: 15 G	PROTEIN: 12 G

INGREDIENTS

- 2 garlic cloves, minced
- 2 medium eggplants, halved
- ¼ tsp salt
- ½ cup plain Greek yogurt
- ¼ tsp pepper
- 3 tbsp olive oil, divided
- 2 cups cooked quinoa
- zest and juice of 1 lemon
- 1 pint cremini mushrooms, quartered
- 1 red onion, diced
- 2 cups kale, torn
- 1 tbsp fresh thyme, chopped
- some lemon wedges, garnish
- 3 tbsp fresh parsley, chopped for garnish

DIRECTIONS

1. Preheat the oven to 400 °F.
2. Add some parchment paper to a baking sheet.
3. Scoop out ⅓ of the eggplant flesh and then rub the inside with 1 ½ teaspoons of oil. Place the eggplant on the baking tray.
4. In a large skillet, add the remaining olive oil and onion and cook for 3–4 minutes over medium heat. Then add the garlic and cook for another minute.
5. Add the mushrooms and cook for 4–5 minutes before adding the quinoa and kale. Cook long enough for the kale to wilt.
6. Season the mixture with salt, pepper, lemon juice, lemon zest, and thyme, then mix.
7. Scoop the mixture into the eggplant and roast them in the oven for 17–20 minutes or until tender. Once done, allow the eggplants to cool for 5 minutes.
8. Serve immediately with some yogurt, lemon wedges, and some parsley.

Easy Mediterranean Pocket Sandwich

This quick and customizable wrap offers the vibrant flavors of the Mediterranean in a modern twist. While not a traditional gyro cooked on a rotisserie, this recipe uses tender, pre-cooked chicken or lamb combined with fresh vegetables and creamy tzatziki, all wrapped in warm pita bread. Perfect for a satisfying meal in no time.

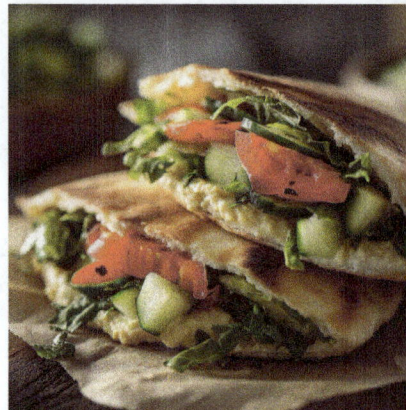

TIME: 10 MIN	SERVINGS: 4	PREP: 10 MIN	COOK: None
CALORIES: 249 KCAL	CARBS: 9.8 G	FAT: 11.1 G	PROTEIN: 27.1 G

INGREDIENTS

- 4 pita breads
- 2 cups cooked chicken or lamb, thinly sliced (rotisserie chicken works well)
- 1 cup lettuce, shredded
- 1 cup tomatoes, diced
- 1 cup cucumbers, diced
- 1 small red onion, thinly sliced
- 1 cup tzatziki sauce (store-bought or homemade

TZATZIKI SAUCE INGREDIENTS

- A refreshing and creamy Greek yogurt-based sauce, perfect for pairing with wraps, grilled meats, or as a dip for vegetables and pita bread.
- 1 cup plain Greek yogurt (unsweetened)
- ½ cucumber, grated and excess water squeezed out
- 2 cloves garlic, minced
- 1 tbsp fresh dill, finely chopped (or 1 tsp dried dill)
- 1 tbsp fresh lemon juice
- 1 tbsp olive oil
- ¼ tsp salt
- ⅛ tsp black pepper

DIRECTIONS

TZATZIKI SAUCE DIRECTIONS:

1. In a bowl, combine the Greek yogurt, grated cucumber, and minced garlic.
2. Stir in the dill, lemon juice, olive oil, salt, & black pepper.
3. Taste and adjust seasoning as needed.
4. Cover and refrigerate for at least 10 minutes to let the flavors meld. Serve chilled as a sauce, dip, or spread.

DIRECTIONS:

1. Warm the pita bread in a skillet or microwave until soft and pliable.
2. Lay each pita flat and spread a generous spoonful of tzatziki sauce in the center.
3. Layer the cooked meat, lettuce, tomatoes, cucumbers, and red onions on top of the sauce.
4. Fold the pita around the filling to create a wrap.
5. Serve immediately and enjoy this fresh and quick Mediterranean meal.

Chicken Penne with Broccoli and Cheese
(Gluten-Free)

Sometimes you want a hearty, pasta-filled lunch. If that's the case, look no further than this chicken penne recipe.

TIME: 38 MIN	SERVINGS: 6	PREP: 10 MIN	COOK: 28 MIN
CALORIES: 272 KCAL	CARBS: 26.4 G	FAT: 11.5 G	PROTEIN: 15.6 G

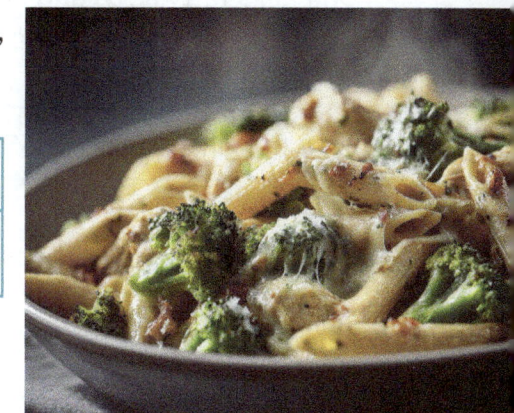

INGREDIENTS

- 1 cup cooked chicken breast, diced into ½-inch pieces
- ½ tsp ground black pepper
- 1 cup gorgonzola, crumbled
- ⅛ cup chicken broth
- 2 cups broccoli florets
- 1 ½ cup cream
- 1 tsp garlic powder
- 1 tbsp rice flour
- 1 tsp salt
- 3 cups pasta, gluten-free

DIRECTIONS

1. Preheat the oven to 350 °F.
2. Add the pasta and 2 quarts of water to a large pot and boil. Cook the pasta for 10 minutes, uncovered. Drain the pasta before tossing it with ½ teaspoon of garlic powder.
3. Fill a new, medium-sized pot with water and boil before adding the broccoli and cook it for 5 minutes. Drain well and add the remaining garlic powder.
4. Add the pasta, chicken, and broccoli to an 8 x 11-inch casserole dish, and mix.
5. In a separate bowl, add ½ a cup of cream with the flour, whisking the lumps out.
6. In a clean skillet, add the broth, pepper, remaining cream, and salt before stirring in the cream mixture. Stir the mixture while it reaches a boil.
7. Lower the heat to allow the sauce to thicken for 5 minutes while still stirring.
8. Add the cheese and continue to stir as the cheese melts. Pour over the casserole's contents.
9. Add a lid to the dish and bake it in the oven for 8 minutes.
10. Remove and serve immediately.

Salmon and Cucumber Bowl

This delicious meal can be thrown together in under an hour and is full of omega-3 fatty acids and fiber. Don't peel the cucumber, as it brings a unique coolness and crunch to this meal.

TIME: 50 MIN	SERVINGS: 4	PREP: 10 MIN	COOK: 40 MIN
CALORIES: 841 KCAL	CARBS: 69 G	FAT: 43 G	PROTEIN: 49 G

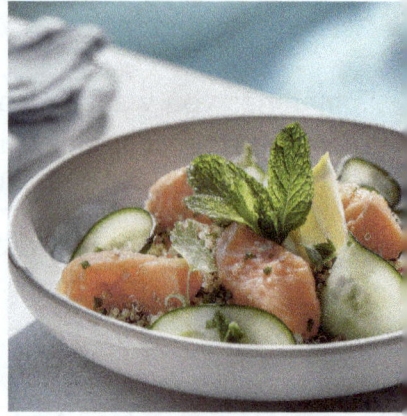

INGREDIENTS

- 2 cups farro
- ¼ cup fresh parsley, chopped
- 4 (6 oz) salmon filets
- ⅓ cup plus 2 tbsp olive oil
- juice of 2 lemons
- ¼ cup seasoned rice vinegar
- ¼ cup fresh dill, chopped
- 1 cucumber, cut into 1-inch chunks
- 2 tbsp Dijon mustard
- ¼ cup fresh mint, chopped
- ¼ tsp pepper
- 1 garlic clove, minced
- ¼ tsp salt

DIRECTIONS

1. Cook the farro in salted boiling water for 25–30 minutes. Drain well.
2. Place the cooked farro in a medium bowl, then add ⅓ cup olive oil, garlic, mustard, and lemon juice before mixing. Season with salt and pepper to taste and set aside.
3. In a different bowl, add the cucumber and lightly smash it with a fork. Pour over the rice vinegar, and then add mint, parsley, dill, salt, and pepper before tossing the contents.
4. Season the fish with salt and pepper before adding the pieces to a skillet over medium heat with olive oil. Cook for 8–10 minutes or until preferred doneness.
5. Break the salmon into bite-sized pieces and serve with the farro and cucumber mixture.

Chicken Salad with Cilantro and Tomatoes
(Gluten-Free + Paleo-Friendly)

With the unique tang that only tomato can bring, the chicken within this dish is sure to pop with flavor. Together with a dash of cilantro, the meal can be enjoyed as is or as a side to a larger meal.

TIME: 35 MIN	SERVINGS: 6	PREP: 35 MIN	COOK: None
CALORIES: 134 KCAL	CARBS: 10.8 G	FAT: 3.6 G	PROTEIN: 15 G

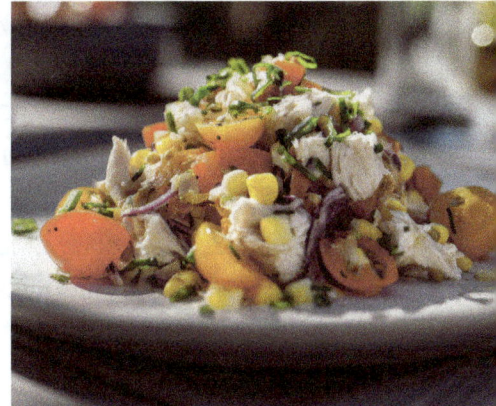

INGREDIENTS

FOR HOMEMADE ITALIAN DRESSING
- ¾ cup olive oil
- ½ tsp crushed red pepper
- 1 tsp lemon juice
- 1 tsp dried basil
- ¼ cup red or white wine vinegar
- ½ tsp onion powder
- ½ tsp pepper
- 1 tsp garlic powder
- 1 tsp dried oregano
- ¾ tsp salt

FOR SALAD:
- 1 cup cherry tomatoes, quartered
- ¼ tsp ground black pepper
- 2 cups cooked chicken, chopped
- ¼ cup cilantro
- 1 green onion sliced
- 1 red chili, seeded and chopped
- 1 cup carrot
- 1 cup medium red bell pepper, chopped
- 1 cup corn
- 3 tbsp Italian dressing

DIRECTIONS

DIRECTIONS FOR SALAD:
1. In a sealable container, add all the ingredients and shake until well-blended.
2. Always give the dressing a shake before use.

DIRECTIONS FOR SALAD:
1. Add the tomatoes, chili, dressing, and black pepper to a blender then purée the mixture. Set this aside.
2. Toss the remaining ingredients in a large bowl.
3. Pour the purée dressing over the salad and toss.
4. Cover the salad with plastic film and allow it to chill for 20 minutes before serving.

Greek Quinoa Bowl
(Gluten-Free)

The Greek quinoa bowl is great as a lunchbox meal that can be served with your choice of colorful peppers, olives, hummus, pita, tomatoes, avocado, or a combination of these ingredients. Explore the different textures and tastes by combining these delightful Mediterranean ingredients.

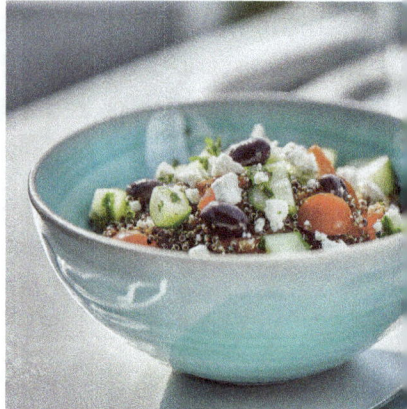

TIME: 17 MIN	SERVINGS: 3	PREP: 12 MIN	COOK: 5 MIN
CALORIES: 440 KCAL	CARBS: 43 G	FAT: 25 G	PROTEIN: 11 G

INGREDIENTS

- ⅓ cup feta cheese, crumbled
- 1 cup quinoa
- ¼ tsp salt
- 1–2 tbsp fresh parsley
- ¼ tsp pepper
- 1 ½ cups water
- ¼ cup olive oil
- 2–3 tbsp apple cider vinegar
- 1 cup red bell pepper, chopped
- 1 cup green bell pepper, chopped

DIRECTIONS

1. For a nuttier taste to your quinoa, add it to a saucepan and toast it with no water for a few minutes before adding the liquid.
2. After adding the water, raise the temperature to high, and bring the saucepan to a boil before reducing the temperature to low. Allow the contents to simmer before adding the lid to cook for 12–13 minutes.
3. Once cooked, fluff the quinoa, add the feta and bell peppers, then mix well. Alternatively, if serving the dish cold, chill the quinoa before adding the cheese and vegetables.
4. In a small bowl, add the olive oil, vinegar, and parsley before whisking and pouring over the quinoa mixture. Toss well.

Spanish Frittata
(Paleo-Friendly + Gluten-Free)

Frittata is a classic Mediterranean dish that can be made in many different ways, and your only limitation is your imagination! Enjoy the Spanish frittata as a hot meal accompanied by some roast potatoes spiced with rosemary or cooled with a side of cucumber salad.

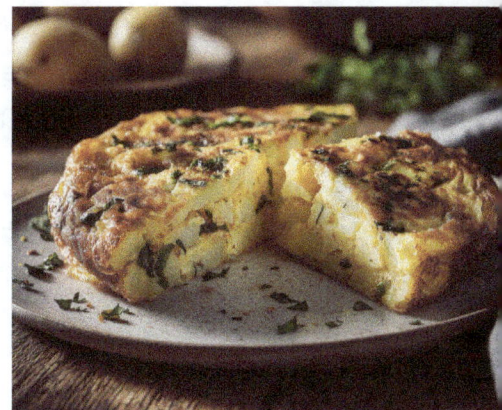

TIME: 40 MIN	SERVINGS: 4	PREP: 8 MIN	COOK: 32 MIN
CALORIES: 182 KCAL	CARBS: 31.5 G	FAT: 2.6 G	PROTEIN: 9.1 G

INGREDIENTS

- 1 medium onion, chopped
- ½ tsp salt
- 6 large eggs
- ¼ tsp ground black pepper
- 2 tsp olive oil
- 1 ½ lbs russet potatoes, peeled and cut into inch-sized cubes

DIRECTIONS

1. Preheat the oven to 400 °F.
2. Add the potatoes to a pot and cover them with water. Raise the temperature to medium-high and cook the potatoes for 15 minutes or until they can be pierced with a fork. Drain and set aside.
3. In a separate bowl, add the salt, pepper, and eggs, and whisk well.
4. Cook the onion in a skillet for 5 minutes, and then add the potatoes.
5. Pour the egg mixture into the potatoes, stir to prevent sticking, and then flatten slightly with a spatula. Keep the heat at medium and continue to cook for another 7 minutes.
6. Place the skillet in the oven and then cook until the egg is set, roughly 5 minutes.
7. Serve as soon as removed from the oven.

Chicken Quinoa Bowl
(Gluten-Free)

Move aside smoothie bowls and make way for quinoa bowls! The pureed pepper sauce adds a hint of spice and a whole lot of flavor to the broiled chicken, while the quinoa brings a unique texture.

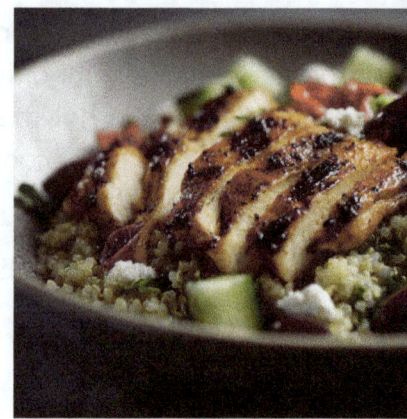

TIME: 30 MIN	SERVINGS: 4	PREP: 12 MIN	COOK: 18 MIN
CALORIES: 519 KCAL	CARBS: 31.2 G	FAT: 26.9 G	PROTEIN: 34.1 G

INGREDIENTS

- 1 cup cucumber, diced
- 1 lb chicken breasts, trimmed
- ¼ cup feta cheese, crumbled
- 1 small clove of garlic, crushed
- 1 (7 oz) jar of roasted red peppers, rinsed
- 4 tbsp olive oil, divided
- ¼ tsp salt
- ¼ cup kalamata olives, pitted and chopped
- 2 cups cooked quinoa
- ¼ cup slivered almonds
- ¼ tsp ground pepper
- ½ tsp ground cumin
- 1 tsp paprika
- ¼ cup red onion, chopped finely
- 2 tablespoons fresh parsley, chopped finely
- ¼ tsp crushed red pepper (optional)

DIRECTIONS

1. Preheat your broiler on high and ensure you place a rack within 3 inches of the heat source.
2. Prepare a baking sheet by lining it with foil.
3. Place the chicken on the baking sheet and add the salt and pepper before adding it to the oven to broil for 14–18 minutes. Turn the meat over once during this time.
4. Remove the chicken from the oven and shred it.
5. Purée the peppers, almonds, cumin, crushed red pepper, 2 tablespoons of oil, paprika, and garlic until smooth and set aside.
6. In a bowl, add the remaining oil, red onion, olives, and quinoa, and mix well.
7. Divide the quinoa and top with cucumber, red pepper sauce, and chicken.
8. Add the crumbled feta and parsley before serving.

Salmon Pita

Not in the mood for a large lunch? Throw together some delicious, cooked salmon, refreshing watercress, and a lemony yogurt dressing to make the ideal light lunch that doesn't take forever to make.

TIME: 5 MIN	SERVINGS: 1	PREP: 5 MIN	COOK: None
CALORIES: 239 KCAL	CARBS: 19 G	FAT: 7.1 G	PROTEIN: 24.8 G

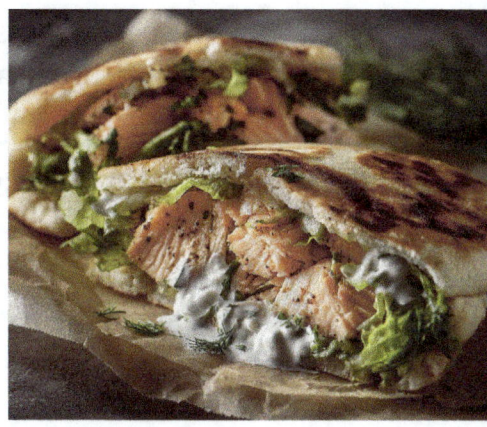

INGREDIENTS

- ½ (6-inch) pita bread, whole-grain
- 2 tbsp plain yogurt
- 3 oz salmon, cooked
- 2 tsp fresh dill, chopped
- 2 tsp lemon juice
- ½ cup watercress
- ½ tsp prepared horseradish

DIRECTIONS

1. Add the yogurt, lemon juice, horseradish, and dill to a bowl and mix before gently stirring in the cooked salmon.
2. Add the watercress to the pita before adding the salmon mixture. Enjoy immediately.

Greek Spanakopita

A flaky and savory Greek spinach pie made with layers of buttery phyllo dough, spinach, and a creamy feta filling.

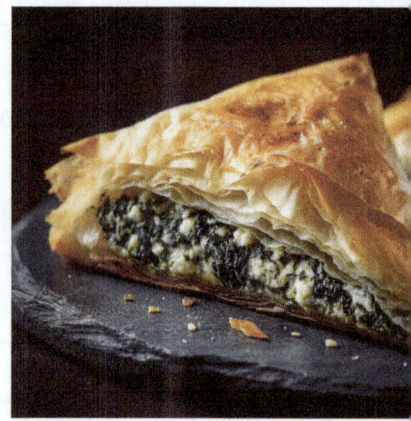

TIME: 1 Hr 10 MIN	SERVINGS: 6	PREP: 20 MIN	COOK: 50 MIN
CALORIES: 290 KCAL	CARBS: 24.4 G	FAT: 18.1 G	PROTEIN: 10.2 G

INGREDIENTS

- 1 tbsp olive oil
- 1 medium onion, finely chopped
- 2 cloves garlic, minced
- 1 lb fresh spinach, washed and chopped
- (or 16 oz frozen spinach, thawed and drained)
- 8 oz feta cheese, crumbled
- 2 eggs, lightly beaten
- ½ cup fresh parsley, chopped
- ½ tsp nutmeg
- ¼ tsp salt
- ¼ tsp pepper
- 1 package phyllo dough, thawed (16-18 sheets)
- ½ cup butter, melted (or olive oil for brushing

DIRECTIONS

1. Preheat the oven to 375°F. Grease a 9x13-inch baking dish with butter or olive oil.
2. **Prepare Filling:**
   - Heat olive oil in a large skillet over medium heat. Sauté the onion and garlic until soft.
   - Add the spinach and cook until wilted (or heated through if using frozen spinach). Remove from heat and let cool.
   - In a mixing bowl, combine the spinach mixture, feta cheese, eggs, parsley, nutmeg, salt, and pepper. Mix well.
3. **Layer Phyllo Dough:**
   - Place a sheet of phyllo dough in the bottom of the baking dish, letting the edges hang over the sides. Brush lightly with melted butter or olive oil.
   - Repeat with 7-8 more sheets, brushing each with butter or oil.
4. **Add Filling & Layers:**
   - Spread the spinach and feta filling evenly over the layered phyllo dough.
   - Layer 8-10 more sheets of phyllo on top of the filling, brushing each with butter or oil. Tuck in the edges of the dough to seal the filling.
   - Using a sharp knife, score the top layer of phyllo into squares or triangles.
5. **Bake & Serve:**
   - Bake for 40-50 minutes, or until the top is golden and crisp.
   - Let the spanakopita cool for 10 minutes before cutting and serving. Enjoy warm or at room temperature.

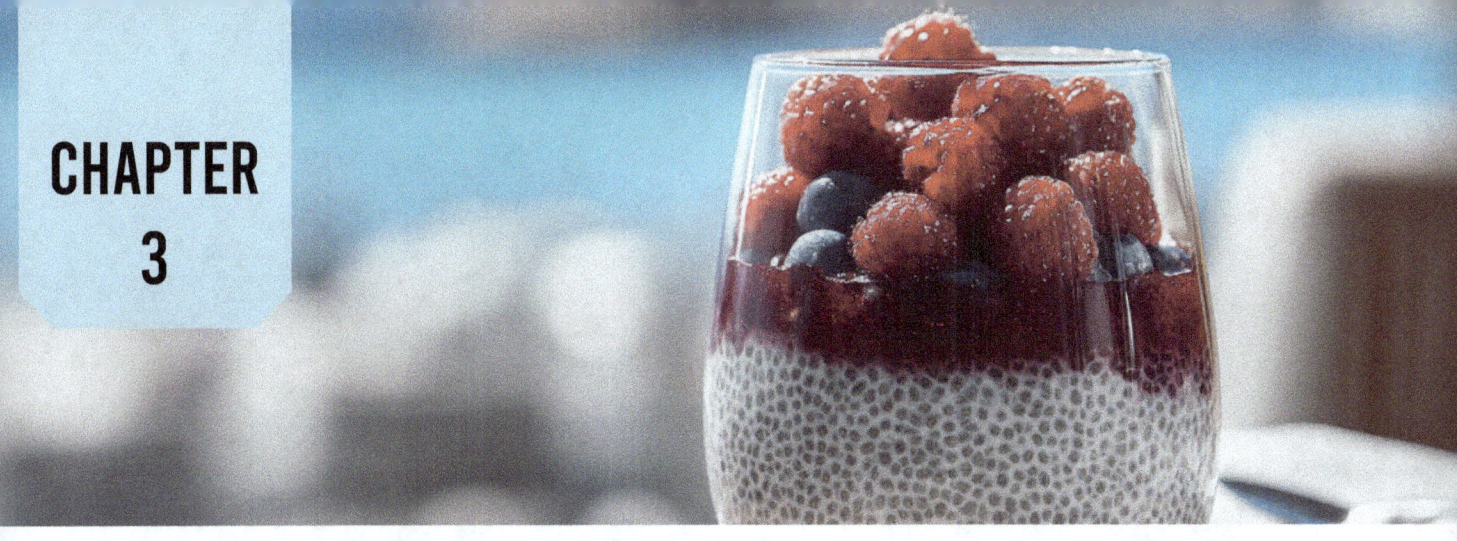

CHAPTER 3

Breakfast and Snacks

Breakfast isn't the most important meal of the day in the Mediterranean. Usually, foods are sampled or snacked on, resulting in light meals instead of the hearty meals reserved for dinner or lunch. In Turkey, people may enjoy a light soup, while in Israel, a tomato and cucumber salad is enjoyed with olive oil-dipped bread. These are only some of the treasures you'll uncover as you explore Mediterranean cuisine.

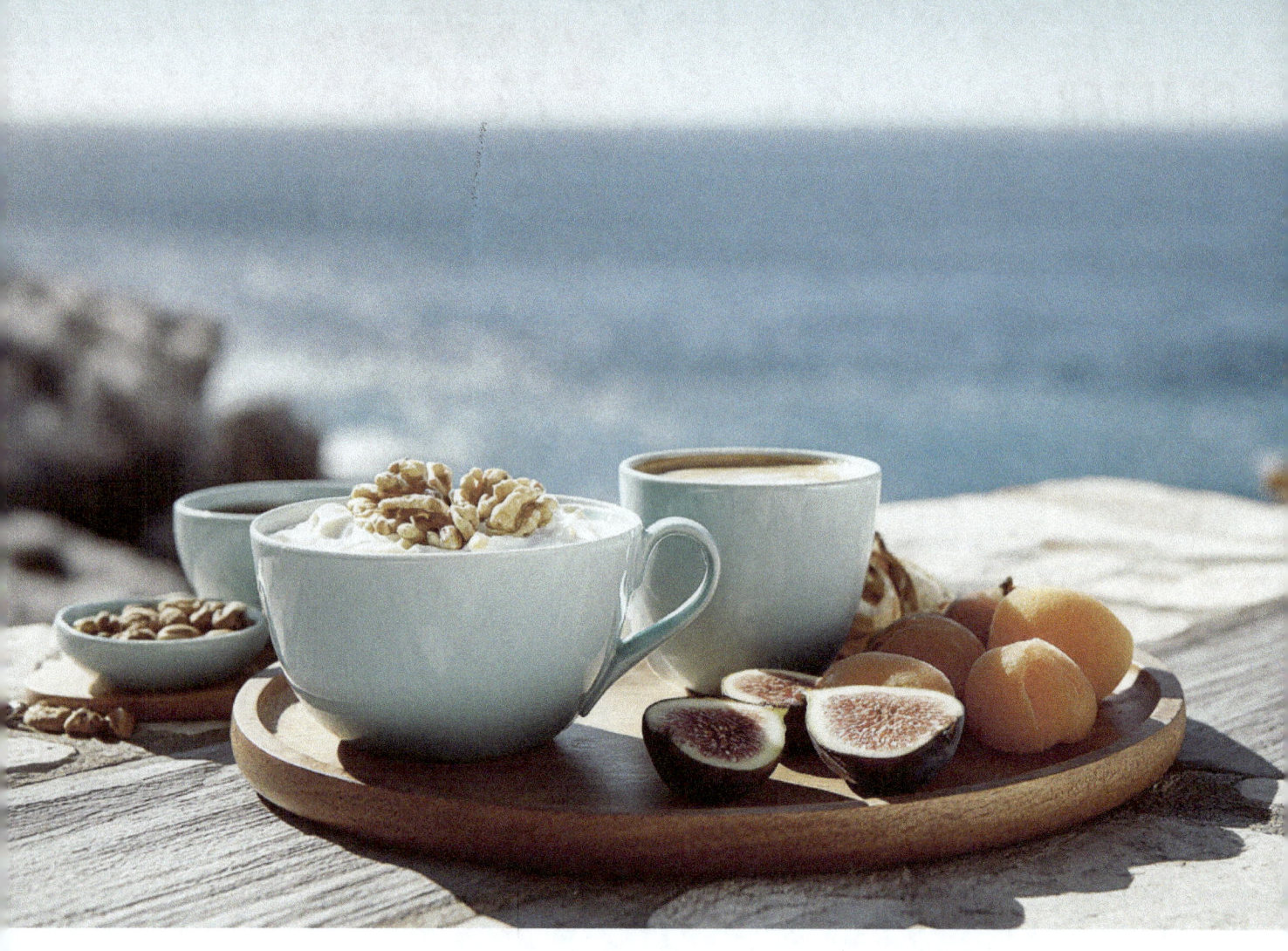

Breakfast
MEDITERRANEAN
Style

Oeufs Brouillés

(French Scrambled Eggs) (Vegetarian-Friendly)

There is such a thing as a perfect egg, and that's oeufs brouillés. These are not just any scrambled eggs, but scrambled eggs made with chilled butter and cooked over a lower temperature while continually stirring. Serve with several slices of crispy baguette slices and top with fresh chives to get the full taste experience.

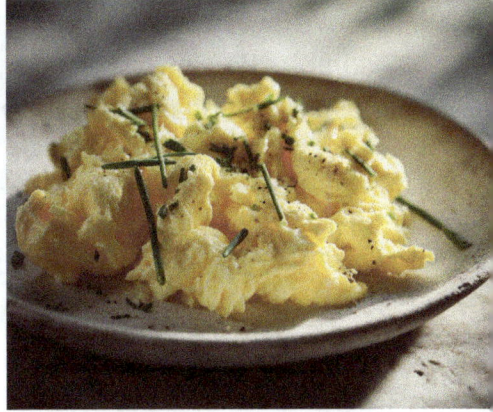

TIME: 26 MIN	SERVINGS: 2	PREP: 8 MIN	COOK: 18 MIN
CALORIES: 393 KCAL	CARBS: 25 G	FAT: 26 G	PROTEIN: 15 G

INGREDIENTS

- 3 eggs, whisked lightly
- 2 tbsp fresh chives, chopped
- 2 tbsp cream
- 1 tbsp butter, chilled and diced
- olive oil for drizzling
- ¼ tsp salt
- ¼ tsp pepper
- 4 baguette slices, toasted

DIRECTIONS

1. Add the chilled butter to the whisked eggs.
2. Pour the eggs into a cold pan before adding them to low heat to cook. Stir continually as the eggs cook.
3. Once half the eggs are set, add the salt, pepper, chives, and cream.
4. Continue to stir and cook until the eggs are completely set but not overcooked.
5. Transfer the eggs onto the toasted baguette slices and drizzle the olive oil over the top before serving.

Muffin Frittatas

(Gluten-Free + Vegetarian-Friendly)

Move over classic frittata! Make way for muffin-sized frittatas! The combination of red pepper, onion, and zucchini makes a tantalizing taste that enhances the subtleness of the mozzarella.

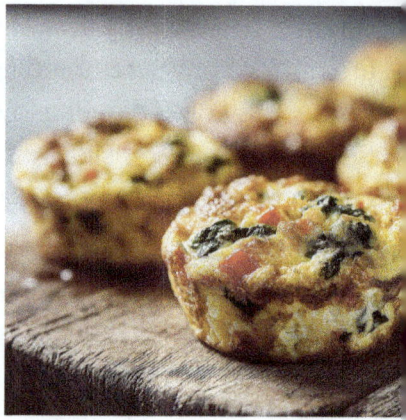

TIME: 30 MIN	SERVINGS: 6 (12 frittatas)	PREP: 10 MIN	COOK: 20 MIN
CALORIES: 164 KCAL	CARBS: 3 G	FAT: 11 G	PROTEIN: 12 G

INGREDIENTS

- ¾ cup zucchini, chopped
- 6 large eggs
- ⅛ tsp pepper
- ¼ cup red bell pepper, chopped
- ¼ tsp salt
- ½ cup milk
- 1 cup mozzarella cheese, shredded
- 2 tbsp red onion, chopped

DIRECTIONS

1. Preheat the oven to 350 °F.
2. In a bowl, whisk the pepper, milk, eggs, and salt together before adding the pepper, onion, zucchini, and cheese.
3. In 12 muffin cups (or a tray with large enough cups), pour ¼ cup of the egg mixture before adding them to the oven to bake for 20 minutes. The egg should be set.
4. Allow the frittatas to cool for 5 minutes before serving.

Mediterranean Sunkissed Granola
(Vegan-Friendly + Vegetarian-Friendly)

Homemade granola gives you the option to add whatever you want to your breakfast granola and control the fat and sugar content. The maple syrup brings with it a natural sweetness, while the nuts bring a delightful crunch. Enjoy with milk, milk alternative, or unsweetened Greek yogurt.

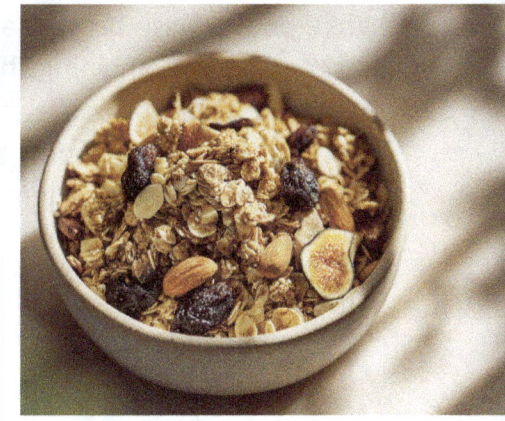

TIME: 1 Hr 20 MIN	SERVINGS: 14 (7 cups)	PREP: 5 MIN	COOK: 1 Hr 15 MIN
CALORIES: 214 KCAL	CARBS: 27.5 G	FAT: 8.8 G	PROTEIN: 5.6 G

INGREDIENTS

- ¼ cup olive oil
- ¼ cup dates, roughly chopped
- 5 cups rolled oats
- ¼ cup dried apricots, roughly chopped
- ¾ cup shredded coconut
- 2 tbsp Grade A maple syrup
- ¼ cup slivered almonds
- ¾ tsp salt
- ¼ cup dried figs, roughly chopped

DIRECTIONS

1. Preheat the oven to 250 °F.
2. Add all the dry ingredients (except for the dried fruit), then the oil, then the syrup (the oil will help to pour the syrup easier), and then mix well.
3. Scoop the granola onto oven pans and even it as much as possible.
4. Add the pans to the oven and bake for 1-¼ hours. Stir the granola every 20 minutes to prevent it from burning.
5. After baking, allow the granola to cool before adding the dried fruit.
6. Mix well and place it in an air-tight container.

Chickpea Hash and Eggs

(Vegetarian-Friendly + Gluten-Free)

While potato hash browns are delicious, why not add to their flavor and texture by combining the potatoes with other vegetables? With the addition of chickpeas, carrots, celery, and onion, your morning hash browns take on a new tantalizing taste. As for the eggs that top the hashbrowns, serve them sunny side up.

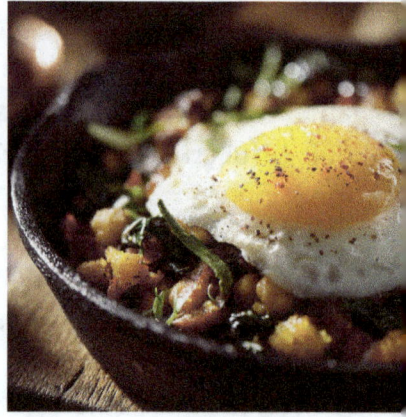

TIME: 30 MIN	SERVINGS: 2	PREP: 10 MIN	COOK: 20 MIN
CALORIES: 475 KCAL	CARBS: 51 G	FAT: 25 G	PROTEIN: 14 G

INGREDIENTS

- ½ medium yellow onion, diced
- 2 large eggs
- 1 tbsp chopped fresh parsley or 1 tsp dried
- 1 (15.5 oz) can of chickpeas, drained, rinsed, and dried
- 3 tbsp olive oil, divided and extra for coating
- 1 carrot, diced
- ½ tsp salt
- 1 garlic clove, minced
- ½ cup low-sodium vegetable stock
- 1 celery stalk, diced
- 2 tsp smoked paprika
- a pinch of black pepper

DIRECTIONS

1. Add 2 tablespoons of oil, salt, and chickpeas to a skillet over medium heat. Don't stir the chickpeas; allow them to brown on 1 side for 5 minutes.
2. Now stir the chickpeas, so the cooked side is up, and cook for a few minutes.
3. Remove the chickpeas, add the parsley and paprika, and stir until well coated.
4. To the same skillet, add the last of the oil, garlic, celery, carrot, and onion before sautéing the vegetables over medium-high until soft.
5. Return the chickpeas and stir together with the vegetables, and add some stock, just enough to cover the bottom part of the pan. Mash the mixture coarsely with a masher.
6. Cook the mixture until most of the stock has cooked away, stirring to keep the mixture moist.
7. In a fresh skillet, coat with olive oil and cook the eggs sunny side up over medium heat for 2 minutes.
8. Add the eggs to the top of the hash and serve immediately.

Fig and Ricotta Overnight Oats
(Gluten-Free + Vegetarian-Friendly)

The creamy ricotta helps to hold back some of the sweetness of the dried figs. At the same time, the almond slivers provide an irresistible crunch to an enjoyable breakfast. Sweeten with a drizzle of honey to bring the whole dish together.

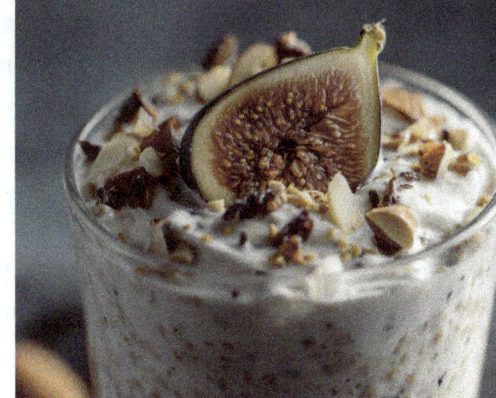

TIME: 8 Hr 5 MIN	SERVINGS: 1	PREP: 5 MIN + 8 Hr Chill	COOK: None
CALORIES: 294 KCAL	CARBS: 47.5 G	FAT: 8.5 G	PROTEIN: 10.4 G

INGREDIENTS

- 2 tbsp ricotta cheese
- ½ cup rolled oats, gluten-free
- 1 tbsp toasted sliced almonds
- ½ cup water
- 2 tsp honey
- 2 tbsp chopped dried figs
- pinch of salt

DIRECTIONS

1. Add the salt, water, and oats in a jar before covering them with plastic cling wrap and leaving it in the fridge till morning.
2. When ready to eat breakfast, heat and top with the remaining ingredients before enjoying.

Mediterranean Egg Muffins
(Vegetarian-Friendly + Gluten-Free)

This is another low-carb breakfast that's easy to make, store, and enjoy whenever you want. Egg muffins are the perfect way to start your day as they are stuffed with the mild sweetness of spinach and peppers, the tanginess of tomatoes, and the savoriness of leek, parmesan, and mozzarella.

TIME: 40 MIN	SERVINGS: 2 (6 muffins)	PREP: 20 MIN	COOK: 20 MIN
CALORIES: 308 KCAL	CARBS: 8.7 G	FAT: 19.4 G	PROTEIN: 24.4 G

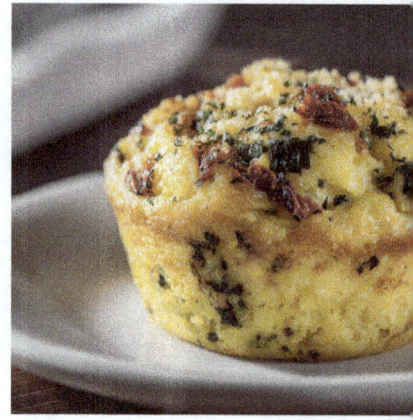

INGREDIENTS

- 3 large eggs
- 0.9 oz mozzarella, shredded
- 2 tbsp milk
- 0.9 oz baby spinach, chopped finely
- 4 tbsp parmesan cheese, grated
- 1 medium tomato, chopped and seeds removed
- 1.2 oz leek, chopped finely
- ¼ medium red pepper, chopped finely
- ¼ tsp pepper
- ¼ tsp salt
- olive oil, coating

DIRECTIONS

1. Preheat the oven to 375 °F.
2. Prepare a 6-cup muffin tin with olive oil.
3. In a bowl, add the parmesan cheese, milk, eggs, and preferred seasoning, then whisk well
4. Use a ladle to pour the egg mixture equally into the muffin cups.
5. Divide the vegetables between the cups and mix well.
6. Add the cheese over the top before adding the muffin tin into the oven.
7. Cook the egg muffins for 15–20 minutes until the egg is set and the cheese is melted.

Berry Chia Pudding
(Vegetarian-Friendly)

Chia seeds are filling and add a crunch and nuttiness that, when combined with the sweetness of the berries in this dessert, make a delightfully light pudding. This dessert can last up to three days in the fridge. However, it's wise to only top with granola once you're ready to serve, or it'll go soggy.

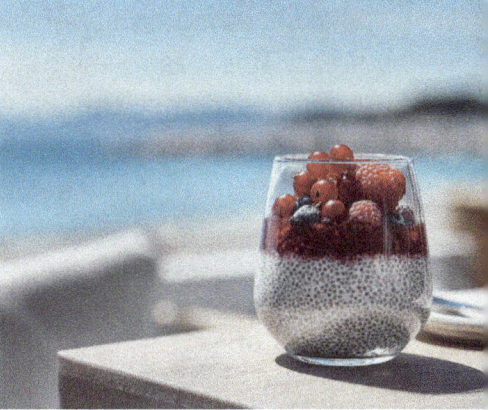

TIME: 8 Hr 5 MIN	SERVINGS: 2	PREP: 5 MIN + 8 Hr Chilling	COOK: None
CALORIES: 343 KCAL	CARBS: 39.4 G	FAT: 15.4 G	PROTEIN: 13.8 G

INGREDIENTS

- ½ cup Greek yogurt
- 1 ¾ cups preferred berries or fruit (can use fresh or frozen), divided
- ¼ cup granola (refer to Homemade Granola recipe)
- 1 cup milk or unsweetened milk alternative
- 1 tbsp pure maple syrup
- ¼ cup chia seeds
- ¾ tsp vanilla extract

DIRECTIONS

1. Take 1 ¼ cups of fruit and milk, and add to a food processor to process until smooth. Pour this mixture into a bowl.
2. Add the syrup, vanilla, and chia seeds in the same bowl, then mix well before covering and adding to the fridge overnight.
3. Split the mixture between 2 bowls before layering equally with the remaining ingredients.

Shakshuka

(Vegetarian-Friendly + Gluten-Free)

Shakshuka is a dish often eaten in North Africa and the Middle Eastern areas. The creamy mixture has earthy and spicy tones thanks to the tomatoes, cumin, paprika, and peppers, making it the perfect dish for breakfast at any time of the year. Enjoyed as is, or you can crumble some feta over it and eat it with a pita.

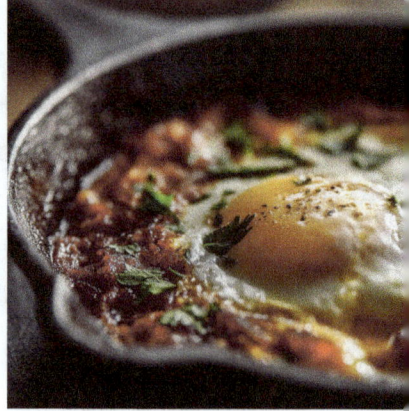

TIME: 30 MIN	SERVINGS: 6	PREP: 10 MIN	COOK: 20 MIN
CALORIES: 146 KCAL	CARBS: 10 G	FAT: 7 G	PROTEIN: 9 G

INGREDIENTS

- 1 medium onion, diced
- 4 garlic cloves, chopped finely
- 1 (28 oz) can of whole peeled tomatoes
- 1 medium red bell pepper, seeded and diced
- 2 tsp paprika
- ¼ tsp chili powder
- 1 small bunch of fresh parsley, chopped
- 1 tsp cumin
- 2 tbsp olive oil
- 6 large eggs
- ¼ tsp pepper
- 1 small bunch of fresh cilantro, chopped
- ¼ tsp salt

DIRECTIONS

1. In a sauté pan, add the olive oil, onion, and bell pepper, and cook for 5 minutes over medium heat.
2. Add the various spices and garlic, and then cook for another minute.
3. Pour the whole can of tomatoes into the pan before breaking them apart with a spoon. Season to taste before bringing the mixture to a simmer.
4. Make 6 wells in the mixture with a spoon before cracking the eggs into them.
5. Add a lid to the pan and allow the mixture to cook until the eggs are done to your preference.
6. Dust with parsley and cilantro before serving.

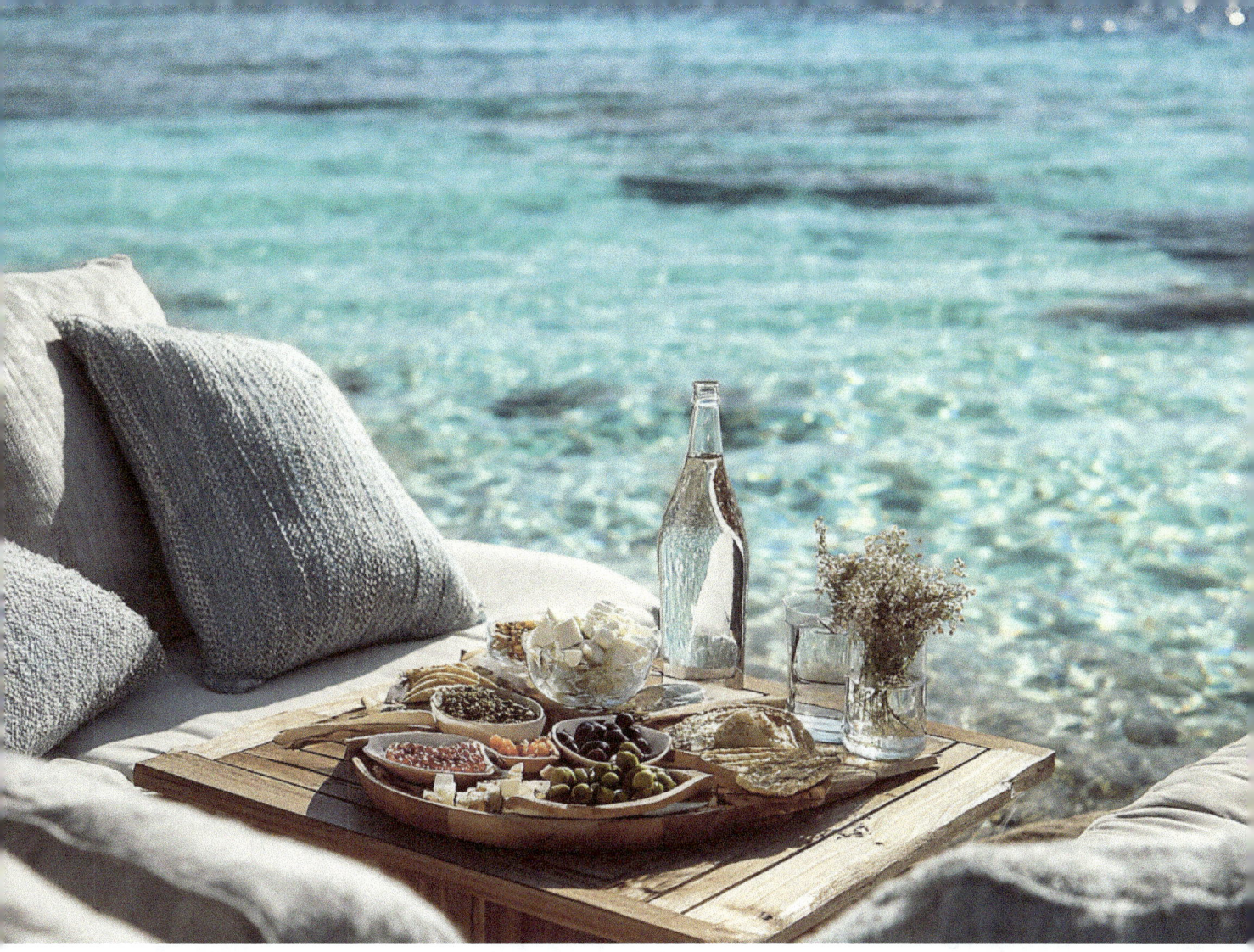

Snacks
MEDITERRANEAN
Style

COOK YOUR BEST LIFE MEDITERRANEAN COOKING RECIPES | 53

No Bake Coconut Cookies
(Keto-Friendly + Gluten-Free)

While not baked cookies, these delightfully low-carb snacks are perfect for protecting you from a snack attack. With only three ingredients, this recipe isn't only easy to make, but the lightness and nuttiness of the coconut will have you coming back again and again, making this your go-to keto snack.

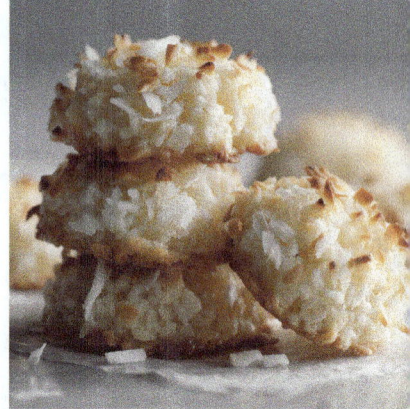

TIME: 5 MIN	SERVINGS: 10	PREP: 5 MIN	COOK: None
CALORIES: 277 KCAL	CARBS: 3.9 G	FAT: 29.7 G	PROTEIN: 0.8 G

INGREDIENTS

- 3 cups dried coconut, plus extra for rolling
- 1 tsp granulated monk fruit sweetener
- 1 cup coconut oil melted

DIRECTIONS

1. Add all the ingredients to a bowl and mix.
2. Wet your hands slightly before dividing the mixture into 10 pieces. Roll each cookie in the crushed coconut and place them in a tray.
3. Place the tray in the fridge and wait until the cookies are firm.
4. Serve immediately or store in the freezer for a few months.

Salmon, Cucumber, and Avocado Bites
(Paleo-Friendly + Gluten-Free)

These tiny bite-sized snacks will soon become your go-to for any dinner party. The crunch of the fresh cucumber is complemented by the creaminess of the freshly made mashed avocado and the saltiness of the smoked salmon.

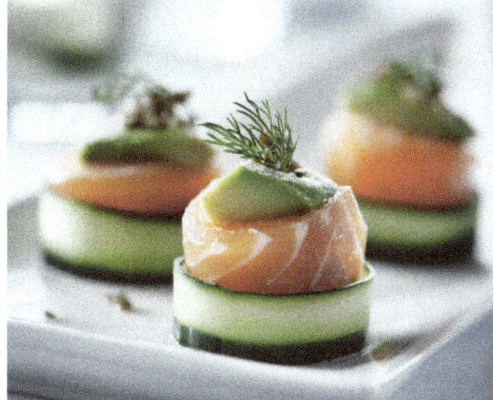

TIME: 10 MIN	SERVINGS: 4 (12 pieces)	PREP: 10 MIN	COOK: None
CALORIES: 46 KCAL	CARBS: 2 G	FAT: 3 G	PROTEIN: 3 G

INGREDIENTS

- 6 oz smoked salmon, sliced thinly
- 1 large avocado, peeled and pitted
- 1 medium cucumber, cut to ¼-inch pieces
- ½ tbsp lime juice
- black pepper, garnish
- chives, garnish

DIRECTIONS

1. Lay the cucumber pieces out on a tray.
2. Mash the avocado and lime in a bowl until smooth.
3. Add a dollop of avocado to the cucumber rounds with some smoked salmon.
4. Add some chives and freshly ground black pepper, then serve immediately.

Chocolate Cupcakes

(Keto-Friendly + Vegetarian-Friendly)

Thanks to coconut flour and monk fruit sweetener, you can create wonderfully light and fluffy chocolate cupcakes without any of the guilt.

TIME: 30 MIN	SERVINGS: 12	PREP: 10 MIN	COOK: 20 MIN
CALORIES: 86 KCAL	CARBS: 4.3 G	FAT: 7.3 G	PROTEIN: 3 G

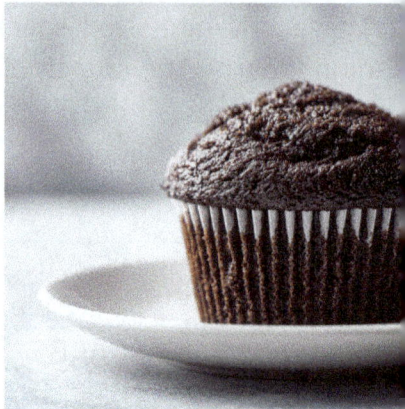

INGREDIENTS

- 1 tsp monk fruit sweetener
- ½ cup almond milk, unsweetened
- ½ cup cacao powder
- 4 large eggs
- 4 tbsp olive oil
- 1 tsp vanilla extract
- ¼ tsp salt
- ½ tsp baking powder
- 1 tsp baking powder
- ⅓ cup coconut flour

DIRECTIONS

1. Preheat the oven to 350 °F.
2. Combine the baking powder, baking soda, cacao powder, salt, and coconut flour, then mix.
3. Create a well in the center of the dry ingredients to add monk fruit sweetener, eggs, olive oil, and almond milk before mixing.
4. Let the mixture sit undisturbed for 5-8 minutes, allowing it to thicken. If it is too thick, add 2 tablespoons of water and stir. Continue until the desired consistency.
5. Place 2 tablespoons of batter in cupcake molds or trays before baking for 20 minutes. An inserted toothpick should come out clean. If not, cook for a further 2 minutes.

Almond Butter Mug Cake

The subtle, creamy flavor of almonds in this cake strikes the perfect balance between satisfying your sweet tooth without overwhelming your taste buds with sugar. Indulge in a guilt-free treat that will leave you feeling fully satisfied.

TIME: 7 MIN	SERVINGS: 1	PREP: 5 MIN	COOK: 2 MIN
CALORIES: 362 KCAL	CARBS: 27 G	FAT: 26.2 G	PROTEIN: 9.9 G

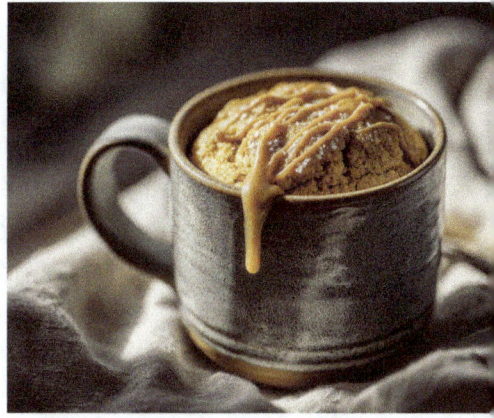

INGREDIENTS

- 2 tbsp coconut flour
- 1 tbsp crushed almonds
- 1 tsp monk fruit sweetener
- 1 tbsp almond butter
- ⅛ tsp baking powder
- 3 tbsp coconut milk

DIRECTIONS

1. Grease a microwave-safe cup with a touch of olive oil.
2. In a bowl, mix all dry ingredients before adding the almond butter and milk.
3. Continue to mix until smooth. If it's too thick, add some milk until the batter is smooth.
4. Gently fold in the nuts.
5. Scoop the mixture into the prepared mug.
6. Microwave the mixture for about 2 minutes. If not fully cooked, cook for a further 30 seconds until done.
7. Cake can be served in a mug, but it will be hot, so be wary.

Mascarpone and Berries Toast
(Vegetarian-Friendly)

Looking for a quick and flavorful snack that's high in fiber? Look no further than mascarpone and berry toast! This delicious treat is more than just a crunchy slice of bread. The combination of tangy mascarpone and sweet, juicy berries creates a delightful balance of sour and sweet flavors. And with the addition of refreshing mint, it's the perfect mid-day snack or a light breakfast to start your day off right.

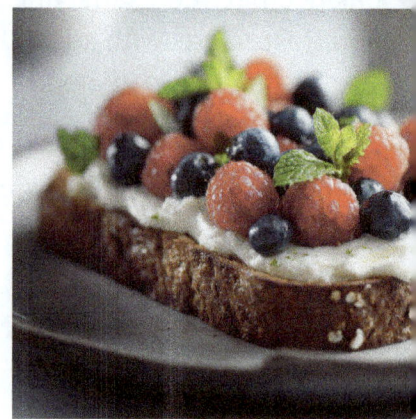

TIME: 5 MIN	SERVINGS: 1	PREP: 5 MIN	COOK: None
CALORIES: 326 KCAL	CARBS: 15.1 G	FAT: 14.2 G	PROTEIN: 7.9 G

INGREDIENTS

- ¼ cup berries of choice
- 1 slice of whole-grain bread, toasted
- 1 tsp fresh mint leaves
- 2 tbsp mascarpone cheese

DIRECTIONS

1. Spread the mascarpone over lightly toasted bread
2. Add a layer the mint and berries, then enjoy.

Yogurt With Blueberries and Honey
(Gluten-Free)

This snack will be on top of your list when you're busy. The honey and berries naturally sweeten the yogurt, so there's no reason to get sweetened yogurt. Even a small drizzle of honey will help enhance the sourness of plain Greek yogurt.

TIME: 5 MIN	SERVINGS: 1	PREP: 5 MIN	COOK: None
CALORIES: 196 KCAL	CARBS: 24.6 G	FAT: 1.1 G	PROTEIN: 23.5 G

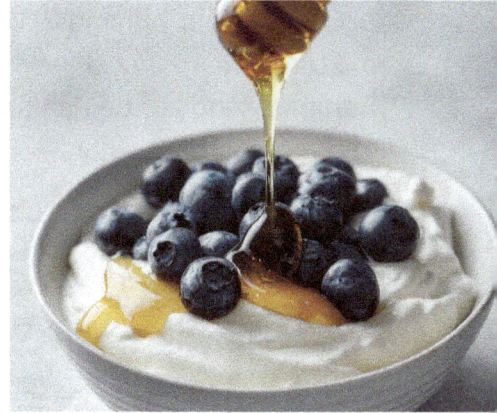

INGREDIENTS

- ½ cup blueberries (or berries of choice)
- 1 cup nonfat plain Greek yogurt
- 1 teaspoon honey

DIRECTIONS

1. Gather ½ cup of blueberries (or other berries), 1 cup of nonfat plain Greek yogurt, and 1 teaspoon of honey.
2. Scoop the Greek yogurt into a small bowl.
3. Drizzle the honey over the yogurt and sprinkle the blueberries on top.
4. Serve and enjoy immediately.

Beet Hummus
(Vegetarian-Friendly, Vegan-Friendly + Gluten-Friendly)

Bored of plain hummus? Well, no more! Add roasted beets to your mixture and enjoy a new flavor with your veggie snacks. While hummus tends to be rich and garlicky, beet hummus is slightly sweet and has a vibrant color.

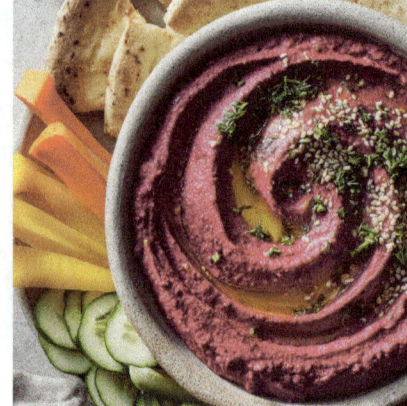

TIME: 10 MIN	SERVINGS: 10 (~2 ⅕ cups)	PREP: 10 MIN	COOK: None
CALORIES: 133 KCAL	CARBS: 9.9 G	FAT: 9.5 G	PROTEIN: 3.3 G

INGREDIENTS
- 1 clove garlic
- 1 (15 oz) can of chickpeas, rinsed
- 1 teaspoon ground cumin
- ¼ cup olive oil
- 8 oz roasted beets, chopped coarsely and patted dry
- ¼ cup lemon juice
- ¼ cup tahini (recipe found in Lettuce Wraps with Tahini Dressing)
- ½ teaspoon salt

DIRECTIONS
1. Add all the ingredients to a blender and process until a smooth consistency is reached.
2. Serve with a side of raw vegetables or pieces of pita.

Sweet and Savory Mezze Platter

Mezze platters are the perfect way to enjoy a variety of Mediterranean flavors while snacking. Enjoy them in combination with pita bread, hummus, tabbouleh, olives and feta cheese for a delicious and healthy snack.

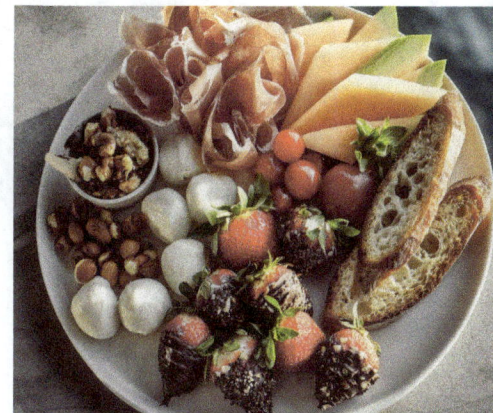

TIME: 10 MIN	SERVINGS: 2 (2 plates)	PREP: 10 MIN	COOK: None
CALORIES: 546 KCAL	CARBS: 44 G	FAT: 33.8 G	PROTEIN: 24 G

INGREDIENTS

- 4 chocolate-dipped strawberries
- 1 cup cubed cantaloupe
- ½ cup unsalted hazelnuts
- 6 thin slices prosciutto, cut in half
- 10 (~ 3.5 oz) small fresh mozzarella balls
- 6 (¼-inch thick) slices of whole-grain baguette
- ½ cup cherry tomato halves

DIRECTIONS

1. Arrange the chocolate-dipped strawberries and cubed cantaloupe on one section of a large serving platter.
2. Place the hazelnuts in a small pile or in a bowl on the platter.
3. Fold the prosciutto slices into loose bundles and arrange them neatly next to the hazelnuts.
4. Add the fresh mozzarella balls to another section of the platter, ensuring they are evenly spaced for easy serving.
5. Arrange the baguette slices near the mozzarella, spreading them slightly for accessibility.
6. Place the cherry tomato halves in a small section or bowl on the platter.

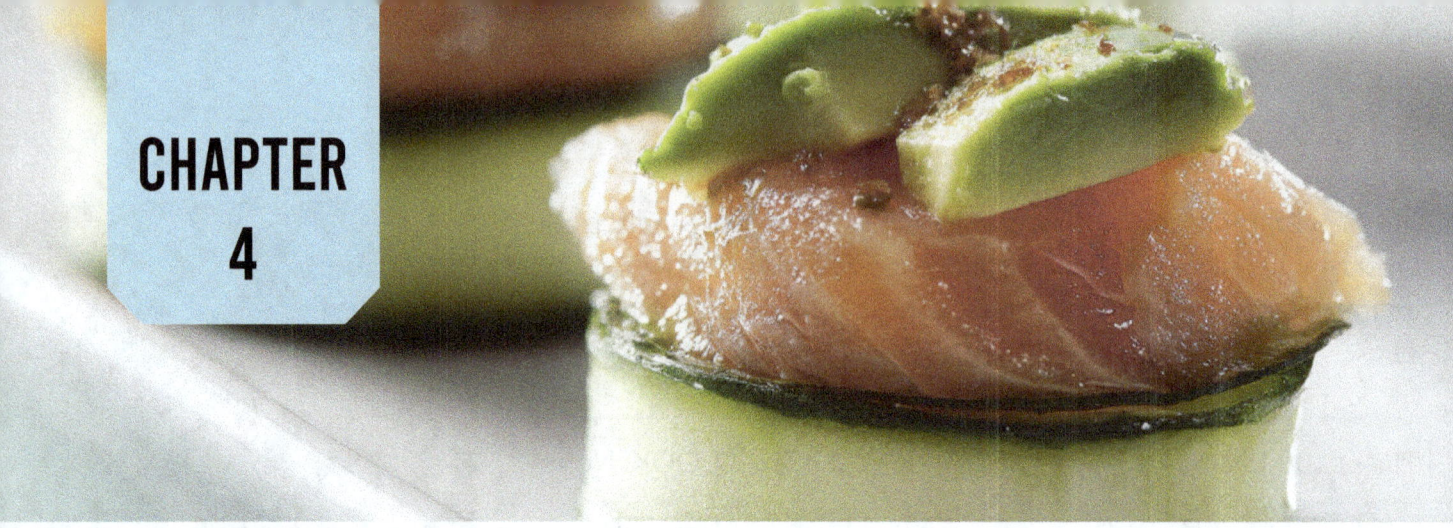

CHAPTER 4

Keto-Friendly
MEDITERRANEAN

If you're on the lookout for some delicious and healthy keto-friendly Mediterranean recipes, we've got you covered. Our selection of recipes will enable you to savor the rich flavors of the Mediterranean while maintaining your keto diet.

Explore our collection of recipes to discover new ways to enjoy the delicious keto-friendly Mediterranean cuisine without sacrificing your health goals.

Here's an overview of the keto diet, along with some helpful tips on preparing yourself for a successful start.

What is the keto diet, and how does it work?

The ketogenic diet is a low-carb diet that encourages using fat as the primary energy source for your body. With this diet, you'll typically consume up to 10% carbohydrates, 20% protein, and 70% fat per day.

As your body adjusts to relying on ketones produced by the breakdown of fats for energy, it's essential to track your ketone levels in blood, urine, or breath to assess how effective your body is at entering and maintaining a state of ketosis. Adjustments to the diet can then be made with guidance from a healthcare professional if needed.

Meal Planning and Preparation

The ketogenic diet isn't the easiest diet to follow, but through proper meal planning and food preparation, it'll be far more manageable! Plus, if you're on a Mediterranean diet already, it's easy to tweak your eating to be more in line with eating keto-friendly by dropping all grains.

Meal planning and preparation are essential for the ketogenic diet to ensure that the meals consumed do not contain high levels of carbs. A meal plan and app can help track macronutrients and prevent accidentally eating more carbs than necessary. If you're using my.Nutiro.com, your customized meal plan for the entire month includes the macronutrients.

Keto Breakfast Muffins

Similar to frittatas, keto breakfast muffins are perfect for all your breakfast needs. The bacon strips create the base of this egg-based, pepper-sweetened, muffin while the spices used can either make it smokey or spicy. The choice is yours. Breakfast muffins are adaptable to your tastes and can last up to 5 days in the fridge.

TIME: 30 MIN	SERVINGS: 6	PREP: 10 MIN	COOK: 20 MIN
CALORIES: 361 KCAL	CARBS: 5 G (1.3 g net carbs)	FAT: 31.8 G	PROTEIN: 14.5 G

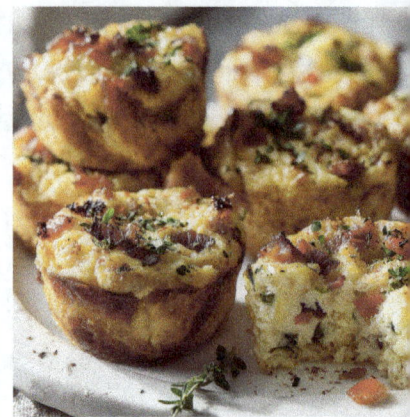

INGREDIENTS

- 1 avocado, smashed
- 2 oz olives, pitted and chopped finely
- 2 tbsp olive oil
- 1 tsp smoked paprika or cayenne pepper
- 9 strips of bacon, each cut in half
- ¼ red bell pepper, julienned
- 6 large eggs
- 2 tbsp fresh thyme
- ¼ cup fresh parsley, chopped (optional)

DIRECTIONS

1. Preheat the oven to 350 °F.
2. Add some olive oil to a 6-muffin tin to grease it.
3. Lay 3 slices of bacon per well to make a cup before cracking an egg into it.
4. Top with a sprinkle of thyme and the julienned bell pepper.
5. Place the muffin tray in the oven and cook for 20 minutes, ensuring the egg is cooked.
6. Remove the muffins from the wells and add some avocado before dusting with paprika or cayenne. Garnish with parsley.

Keto-Friendly Frittata

Frittatas can be made for any diet and still remain in line with the Mediterranean diet. With rich avocado oil and just a hint of tangy garlic, you'll need no more than just a skillet to create a delicious one-pan meal. Don't forget to crumble over the feta before serving.

TIME: 24 MIN	SERVINGS: 2	PREP: 12 MIN	COOK: 12 MIN
CALORIES: 126 KCAL	CARBS: 2.5 G (1.3 g net carbs)	FAT: 9.3 G	PROTEIN: 8.5 G

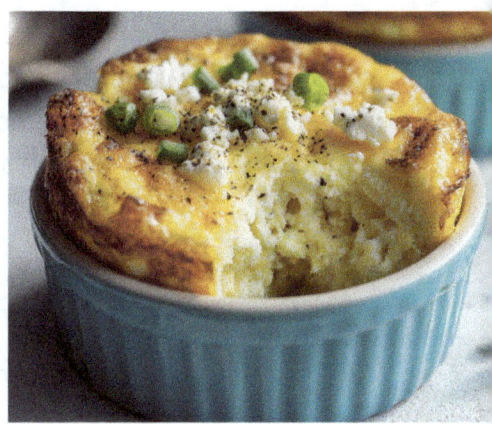

INGREDIENTS

- 4 tbsp feta cheese, crumbled
- 1 green onion
- 1 tbsp avocado oil
- 1 tsp garlic minced
- 2 large eggs
- 1 pinch salt
- 1 pinch ground black pepper

DIRECTIONS

1. Place a skillet over medium heat and add the olive oil.
2. Cook the garlic and onion until translucent and tender.
3. In a medium bowl, add the eggs, 3 tablespoons of feta, pepper, and salt, then whisk well.
4. Pour the egg mixture into the skillet and cook covered until the eggs are almost set.
5. Add the last tablespoon of feta before covering the skillet, allowing the eggs to cook a further few minutes until set.

Mediterranean Branzino

Known as the "Greek Sea Bass," branzino is a mild and flaky fish that can take on a world of flavor when cooked just right. By stuffing the inside of each fish with lemon, oregano, and rosemary, you'll truly get a mouthful of the Mediterranean with each bite that you take.

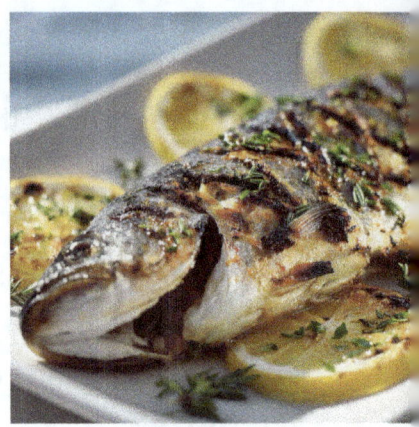

TIME: 40 MIN	SERVINGS: 4	PREP: 15 MIN	COOK: 25 MIN
CALORIES: 380 KCAL	CARBS: 7 G (2 g net carbs)	FAT: 13 G	PROTEIN: 53 G

INGREDIENTS

- ½ cup white wine
- 2 tbsp olive oil, divided
- ¼ tsp pepper
- ¼ cup Italian flat-leaf parsley, chopped
- ¼ tsp salt
- 1 red onion, chopped
- 2 sprigs of fresh rosemary
- 1 tbsp fresh oregano leaves
- ¼ cup lemon juice
- 2 whole Branzino fish, cleaned
- 4 lemon wedges, divided

DIRECTIONS

1. Preheat the oven to 325 °F.
2. In a large baking pan, add the red onion and drizzle a tablespoon of olive oil over it. Season with salt and pepper and mix well.
3. Stuff each fish cavity with a lemon wedge, rosemary sprig, and some red onion. To open the fish, make an incision along the underside from gills to tail, cutting through ribs and flesh, then gently pry it open.
4. Pour the lemon juice and wine over the contents of the pan and dust with oregano.
5. Add a tablespoon of oil over the fish and add to the oven to bake for 25 minutes, or until the fish becomes opaque and a fork can easily flake it.
6. Debone the fish by placing a spatula between the flesh and bones and remove all the bones.
7. Serve both fish on a platter with the remaining lemon wedges and garnish with parsley.

Mediterranean Grilled Swordfish

Swordfish is a mild, white-fleshed fish that is perfect for grilling! Together with a marinade made with olive oil, paprika, cumin, and coriander, the swordfish comes alive with the coastal flavors of Spain.

TIME: 27 MIN	SERVINGS: 4	PREP: 15 MIN	COOK: 8 MIN
CALORIES: 398 KCAL	CARBS: 3.1 G (0.4 g net carbs)	FAT: 30.7 G	PROTEIN: 28.4 G

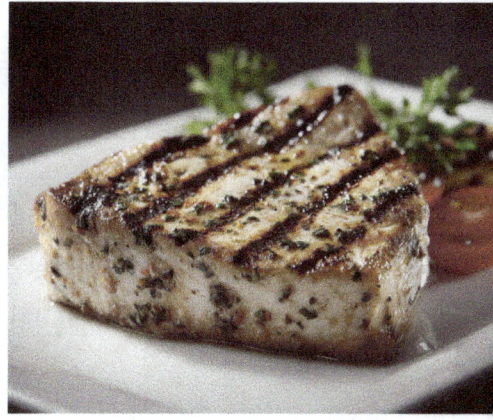

INGREDIENTS

- ½–1 tsp sweet Spanish paprika or smoked paprika
- 4 (5–6 oz) swordfish steaks, inch thick
- ⅓ cup virgin olive oil
- 1 tsp coriander
- ¾ tsp cumin
- 2 tbsp fresh lemon juice, more for later
- ¾ tsp salt
- 6–12 garlic cloves, peeled
- ½ tsp freshly ground black pepper
- crushed red pepper (optional)

DIRECTIONS

1. Add all the spices, garlic, olive oil, and lemon juice to a food processor and blend until smooth and thick.
2. Add the dry-patted swordfish steaks to a pan and pour the marinade over them. Ensure to get the marinade on all sides of the steaks.
3. Set aside the steaks to marinate until the gas grill is heated.
4. Preheat the grill to high, and once ready, add the steaks and cook for 5 minutes before flipping them and cooking for another 3 minutes. The swordfish should remain firm but flake easily.
5. Before serving, add a dash of lemon juice and some red pepper flakes if you want some bite to your dish.

If swordfish isn't available or you're looking for an alternative, here are three excellent options:
1. Halibut
2. Mahi-Mah
3. Tuna Steaks

These fish have a firm texture and mild flavor, making them ideal for grilling and perfect for soaking up the bold Mediterranean marinade in this recipe. Understanding their unique qualities can help you choose the best substitute for your taste and cooking needs.

Mediterranean Chicken Salad

The combination of olives, feta, chicken, and greens, brings many unique flavors together in a salad that will soon become an all-time favorite.

TIME: 20 MIN	SERVINGS: 2	PREP: 5 MIN	COOK: 15 MIN
CALORIES: 628 KCAL	CARBS: 20.8 G (3.3 g net carbs)	FAT: 43.6 G	PROTEIN: 39 G

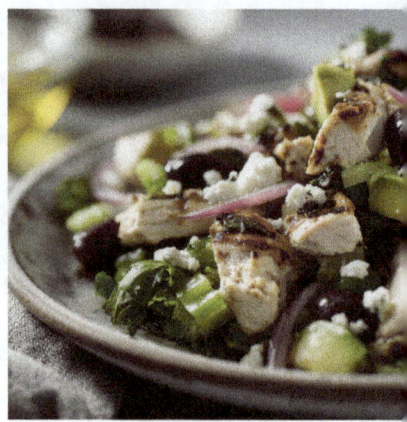

INGREDIENTS

- 1 avocado, chopped
- 8 oz chicken thighs
- 1 oz feta, crumbled
- 1 oz Kalamata olives, pitted
- 4 cups fresh greens
- 1 cup celery, chopped finely
- 2 tbsp avocado oil mayonnaise
- ¼ cup red onion, chopped finely
- ¼ tsp pepper
- ¼ tsp salt

DIRECTIONS

1. Start by cooking the chicken thighs until the juices runs clear when the meat is cut, roughly 15 minutes.
2. While the chicken is cooking, prepare the avocado, celery, and red onions, and add them to a bowl.
3. Cut the chicken into cubes and add to the avocado mixture before adding the avocado oil mayonnaise.
4. Mix the ingredients well before seasoning to taste.
5. In a serving dish, add the mixed greens before adding the chicken salad, feta, and olives before serving.

Chicken and Pesto Zoodles

Pasta is a Mediterranean staple, but zoodles (spiralized zucchini) are a great alternative. Combined with creamy avocado and mild chicken, this dish is filling and flavorful without the pasta.

TIME: 25 MIN	SERVINGS: 1	PREP: 10 MIN	COOK: 15 MIN
CALORIES: 691 KCAL	CARBS: 15.4 G (3.9 g net carbs)	FAT: 56 G	PROTEIN: 37.3 G

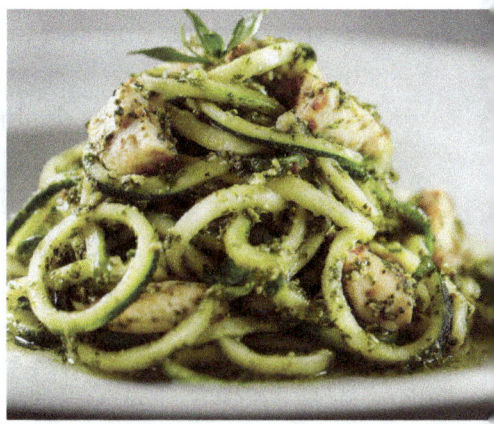

INGREDIENTS

- ½ avocado
- 1 zucchini
- ¼ cup water
- 4 oz chicken breasts
- ¼ cup fresh basil
- 1 tbsp coconut oil
- 1 tbsp olive oil
- 1 pinch ground black pepper
- 1 pinch salt

DIRECTIONS

INSTRUCTIONS FOR ZOODLES:

1. **Wash and Prep the Zucchini:**
   - Rinse the zucchini thoroughly under cold water and pat dry. Trim off the ends.
2. **Create the Noodles:**
   - If using a **spiralizer,** secure the zucchini and turn the handle to create long, spiral-shaped noodles.
   - If using a **julienne peeler,** run it along the zucchini lengthwise to create thin strips.
   - For a **mandoline,** use the julienne attachment to slice the zucchini into noodles.
3. **Optional Cooking:**
   - For raw zoodles: Use them as-is in salads or cold dishes.
   - For cooked zoodles: Heat a large skillet over medium heat, add a drizzle of olive oil, and sauté the zoodles for 2–3 minutes, tossing gently, until just tender. Avoid overcooking to prevent sogginess.

DIRECTIONS:

1. Place a pan over medium heat and add the coconut oil.
2. Add the chicken to the pan and cook thoroughly.
3. As the chicken is cooking, spiralize the zucchini. Alternatively, you can use a hand peeler.
4. Make the cream sauce by adding the remaining ingredients to a blender and blend until well combined.
5. Add the cooked chicken to the zoodles before pouring over the avocado cream sauce.
6. Mix the contents before serving.

Stuffed Avocados

Creamy avocado boats stuffed with tenderly spiced chicken, cream cheese, and sun-ripened tomatoes is a dish well worth trying if you're a little peckish. A light dusting of Parmesan cheese wraps up the dish nicely as it melts ever so slightly in the oven before serving. Great as a meal for one or split between two people with a Greek salad to share.

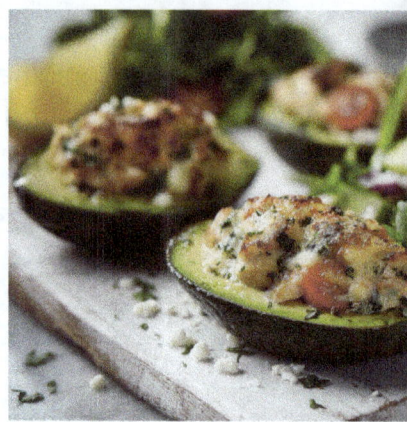

TIME: 45 MIN	SERVINGS: 1	PREP: 20 MIN	COOK: 25 MIN
CALORIES: 1071 KCAL	CARBS: 33.2 G (9.3 g net carbs)	FAT: 88.2 G	PROTEIN: 44.8 G

INGREDIENTS

FOR STUFFED AVOCADOS:
- 2 tbsp parmesan cheese
- 1 avocado
- 3 oz chicken breasts, cooked and shredded
- ¼ cup tomato, chopped
- 1 oz cream cheese
- ¼ tsp pepper
- ¼ tsp salt

FOR GREEK SALAD:
- 3 tbsp crumbled feta cheese
- 2 cups romaine lettuce, cut into small pieces
- 2 tbsp chopped red onions
- 6 cherry tomatoes, cut in half
- 8 slices pickled and jarred banana peppers
- 8 Kalamata olives, pitted and sliced

FOR GREEK SALAD DRESSING:
- ⅛ tsp salt
- ⅛ tsp dried oregano
- 1 tbsp red wine vinegar
- 1 tbsp olive oil
- 1 minced garlic clove (optional)

DIRECTIONS

FOR GREEK SALAD:
1. Add all the ingredients for the salad dressing in a small bowl and whisk until well combined. Set aside.
2. In a large bowl, add the salad ingredients and then drizzle the salad dressing over before tossing. Place in the fridge until ready to serve.

FOR AVOCADOS:
1. Preheat the oven to 400 °F.
2. Shred the chicken and set it aside.
3. Cut the avocado in half, lengthwise, then remove the pit.
4. Scoop out some of the avocado.
5. Place this extra avocado in a bowl with the cooked chicken, tomatoes, and cream cheese before mixing and seasoning to taste.
6. Split the contents between the 2 avocado halves—don't be afraid to scoop out more avocado if needed.
7. Top with the parmesan cheese and place the avocado halves on a baking tray before adding them to the oven.
8. Bake for about 10 minutes to melt the parmesan cheese, and serve hot.

One Skillet Greek Isle Chicken

Creating an entire meal within one skillet doesn't only make cooking much easier, but also quicker to clean up afterward. The nutty artichoke hearts and chicken seasoned to perfection make for a well-rounded dish that's perfect for even the coldest and rainiest of days. Enjoy immediately or freeze for later use, either way will result in a tantalizing meal.

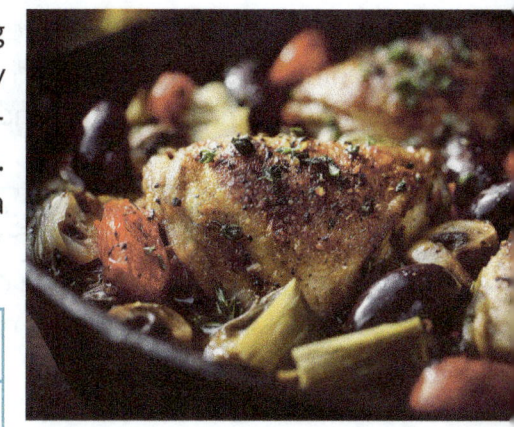

TIME: 30 MIN	SERVINGS: 4	PREP: 15 MIN	COOK: 15 MIN
CALORIES: 474 KCAL	CARBS: 14.5 G (8.7 g net carbs)	FAT: 27.5 G	PROTEIN: 43.1 G

INGREDIENTS

- 1.4 oz spinach
- 8 oz white button mushrooms, sliced
- 1 ½ lbs chicken breasts, cut into 1-inch pieces
- ½ lemon, juiced
- 2 tbsp olive oil
- ⅓ cup kalamata olives
- 1 cup cherry tomatoes
- 1 ½ tbsp Greek seasoning
- 4 garlic cloves, minced
- ½ lemon, sliced
- 14 oz can artichoke hearts
- 1 tsp sea salt
- ½ cup yellow onion, diced
- 2 tbsp basil, chopped, garnish
- 4 tbsp extra virgin olive oil, garnish

DIRECTIONS

1. In a large skillet, heat the oil over medium-high and add the chicken with Greek seasoning (oregano, garlic, onion and a touch of mint) and salt. Like any other spice blend, Greek seasoning can be purchased in bottle form. Cook for roughly 5–7 minutes, and set aside.
2. In the same pan, add the garlic and onion to cook for a minute.
3. Add the lemon slices (keep some for garnishing), lemon juice, olives, artichokes, mushrooms, and tomatoes, then cook until the mushrooms start softening.
4. Return the chicken to the pan before tossing the contents, and then add the spinach. Cook just long enough to wilt the spinach.
5. Before serving the hot dish, garnish with olive oil, lemon slices, and chopped basil.

Seafood Stew

This flavorful seafood stew brings the vibrant scents of the Mediterranean to your kitchen with mussels, shrimp, and a savory blend of tomatoes, garlic, and herbs. Perfect for a cozy meal!

TIME: 30 MIN	SERVINGS: 1	PREP: 10 MIN	COOK: 20 MIN
CALORIES: 175 KCAL	CARBS: 8 G (0.9 g net carbs)	FAT: 7.2 G	PROTEIN: 18.5 G

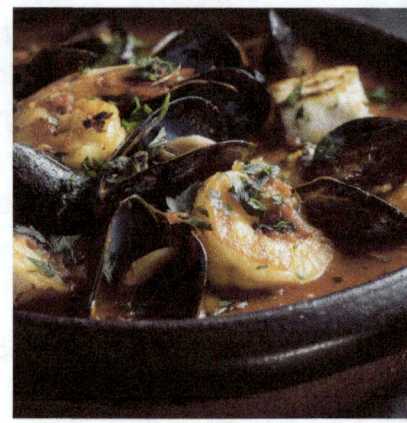

INGREDIENTS

- 1 tbsp olive oil
- 1 small onion, chopped finely
- 5 oz mussels, cleaned
- ¼ pound large shrimp, cleaned and peeled
- a pinch of dried oregano
- ½ tsp sea salt
- 2 garlic cloves, minced
- ½ red bell pepper, chopped
- 1/2 can of diced tomatoes
- 2 cups of fish or chicken stock
- Fresh parsley or cilantro for garnish

DIRECTIONS

1. Heat the olive oil in a large pot over medium heat until it caramelizes. Add the onion and cook until softened.
2. Add the garlic and red bell pepper and cook for another minute.
3. Pour in the canned tomatoes and stock. Bring to a simmer.
4. Add in the seafood and cook until it is all cooked through (about 5 minutes).
5. Season with salt and pepper to taste.
6. Serve hot with fresh parsley or cilantro on top.
7. Season to taste and serve.

Tuscan Garlic Chicken

While the chicken brings its mild flavor to the dish, it's the garlicky undertones with a rich cream base that will have you returning time and time again to sip at the bubbling meal as it cooks. Enjoy over some freshly baked keto-friendly bread, or quickly heat up some zoodles to accompany the hot dish. For directions on how to make zoodles refer to the chicken and zoodles with pesto.

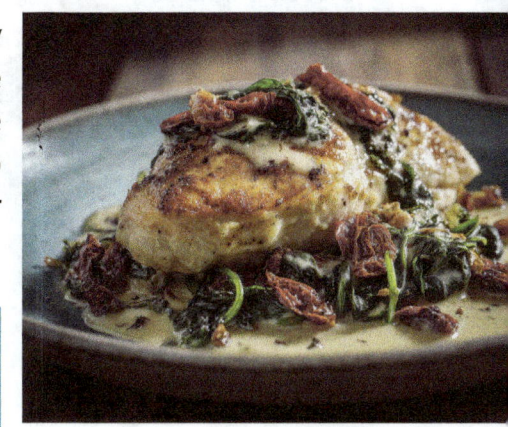

TIME: 250 MIN	SERVINGS: 6	PREP: 10 MIN	COOK: 15 MIN
CALORIES: 368 KCAL	CARBS: 7 G (4 g net carbs)	FAT: 25 G	PROTEIN: 30 G

INGREDIENTS

- 1 ½ pounds chicken breasts, sliced thinly
- 1 tsp Italian seasoning
- 1 cup heavy cream
- ½ cup parmesan cheese
- 2 tbsp olive oil
- 1 tsp garlic powder
- ½ cup sun-dried tomatoes
- 1 cup spinach, chopped
- ½ cup chicken broth

DIRECTIONS

1. Add the chicken and olive oil to a large skillet and cook the meat until it's browned on both sides and not pink in the center. Set aside.
2. In the same skillet, pour in the heavy cream, parmesan cheese, chicken broth, Italian seasoning, and garlic powder, then turn the heat to medium-high. Whisk the mixture until it starts to thicken.
3. Add the tomatoes and spinach to the mixture and allow it to simmer until the greens wilt.
4. Return the chicken to the pan before serving it with keto-friendly pasta or bread.

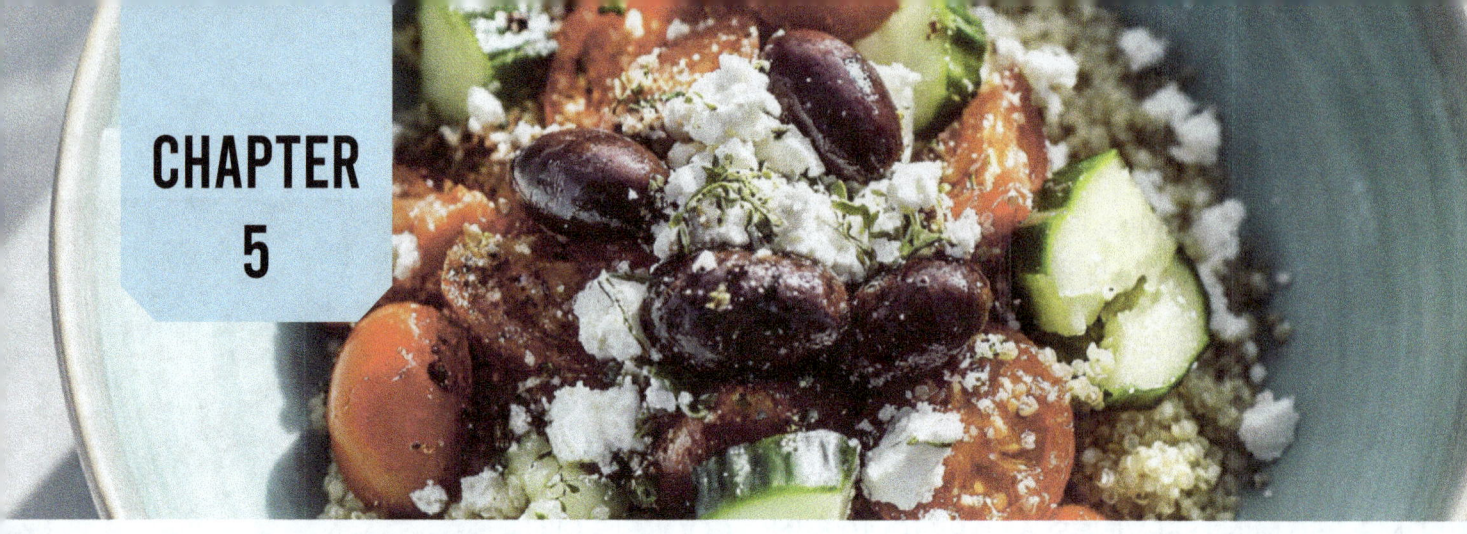

CHAPTER 5

Gluten-Friendly
MEDITERRANEAN

Many people take for granted that they can eat anything, anywhere, anytime. If you're someone who deals with Celiac disease, gluten sensitivity, wheat allergy, or you have Gluten ataxia (the autoimmune disorder), you're aware of the nightmare anything containing gluten can cause in your life.

Gluten is a protein found in wheat, rye, triticale (a wheat-rye hybrid), bulgar, and oats through cross-contamination with other gluten-heavy grains. Gluten can be found in most baked goods, pasta, and even some sauces that use wheat as a thickening agent.

People who get ill from ingesting gluten need to constantly be vigilant with what they eat, as even some cross-contamination with gluten in a kitchen can result in a painful few days. The only sure way to avoid gluten is to prepare your food or thoroughly read the nutritional information on any ready-made meals.

The following recipes will ensure you never miss gluten again, regardless of your reason for eating gluten-free. With an array of grains containing no gluten, flavorful stews, and skillet meals, these Mediterranean treats will provide you to eat the way you want.

Meal Planning and Preparation

Unlike the keto diet, which is very specific with what you can't eat, if you're eating a gluten-free diet, you only need to avoid grains that contain gluten. Other than that, you can prepare your meals the same way as you would on a standard Mediterranean diet.

This diet is only challenging if you don't do your homework about what grains contain gluten. To help you determine what grains and flours you can use, here is a handy list to take with you when you go shopping:

- Quinoa
- Hominy
- Almond
- Amaranth
- Buckwheat
- Corn
- Flax
- Tapioca
- Polenta
- Rice
- Teff
- Sorghum
- Millet
- Soy
- Oat
- Coconut
- Chickpea

If you still want to enjoy the taste of baked goods, you will need to read the packaging to ensure that the food is truly gluten-free or not. However, you'll likely need to give up processed foods or be prepared to spend a little more money to ensure you only get gluten-free food when shopping.

Something that can be a problem with gluten-free diets is that people tend to get constipated due to not getting enough fiber (Raman & Link, 2022). You must increase the number of vegetables you eat or ensure that you eat enough gluten-free grains to make up for the loss of fiber. This is especially true if skipping pasta and bread.

Whether you are going gluten-free because of sensitivities, or allergies, or you want to drop wheat, the best way to get a head start is to collect gluten-free recipes and build a shopping list. Concentrate on gluten-free pasta and bread, the previously mentioned grains, Mediterranean fruits and vegetables, legumes, lean meats, and unsweetened dairy products (Anderson, 2020). Pay close attention to food and beverage options because gluten may be a thickening agent.

Quinoa Salad

Quinoa has a slightly chewy texture with a nutty undertone that melds well with the flavor of pine nuts. Toss together with roasted red bell pepper, onions, and tomato will bring the true taste of the Mediterranean to any mealtime. Don't forget to add the feta for the creamy finish or the fresh basil to the dish. Enjoy as is or with some gluten-free pita bread or avocado.

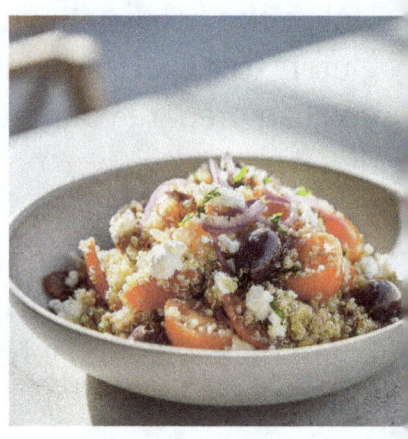

TIME: 25 MIN	SERVINGS: 6	PREP: 15 MIN	COOK: 10 MIN
CALORIES: 359 KCAL	CARBS: 34 G	FAT: 21 G	PROTEIN: 9 G

INGREDIENTS

- 1 clove garlic, minced
- 2 cups multicolored cherry tomatoes, halved
- 3 tbsp red-wine vinegar
- 1 medium red bell pepper, cut into 1-inch pieces
- ¼ cup pine nuts, toasted
- ½ tsp ground pepper, divided
- 1 tbsp fresh oregano, chopped
- 1 cup red onion, sliced
- ¾ cup feta, crumbled
- ¼ cup virgin olive oil, divided
- 4 cups cooked quinoa, cooled
- ¼ cup kalamata olives, pitted
- ¼ tsp salt
- chopped fresh basil for garnish

DIRECTIONS

HOW TO COOK QUINOA

1. Rinse quinoa in a fine-mesh strainer to remove bitterness.
2. Optional: Toast quinoa in a dry saucepan over medium heat for 2–3 minutes.
3. Add 2 cups water or broth and a pinch of salt. Bring to a boil.
4. Reduce heat, cover, and simmer for 15 minutes.
5. Remove from heat, let sit for 5 minutes, then fluff with a fork.

DIRECTIONS:

1. Place a rack within 6 inches of the oven's heat source, and preheat to broil.
2. In a small bowl, add the salt, garlic, and oregano before pouring in 3 tablespoons of oil and ¼ teaspoon of pepper. Whisk the vinaigrette and set it aside.
3. In a larger bowl, add the remaining pepper and oil with the olives, bell pepper, onion, and tomatoes, then toss until well-coated.
4. Transfer the mixture to a rimmed baking sheet, and spread it out. Broil for 8–10 minutes or until the vegetables are lightly charred. Be sure to stir roughly 5 minutes in to ensure even cooking.
5. Remove the vegetables from the pan and discard any juices.
6. Mix the vegetables, pine nuts, feta, and quinoa in a large bowl and drizzle the vinaigrette over the top. Toss gently and serve.

Mediterranean Egg Bowl

There is no need for bacon when you try this savory breakfast. Scrambled eggs with creamy feta go well with any color bell pepper and are accompanied by the peppery aftertaste of the fresh scallions. You don't need to add extra salt because the olives bring a salty flavor to the egg bowl. It is so filling that bread won't even be missed.

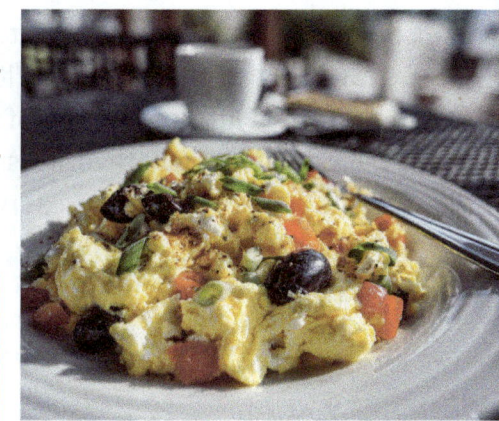

TIME: 10 MIN	SERVINGS: 1	PREP: 5 MIN	COOK: 5 MIN
CALORIES: 346 KCAL	CARBS: 11 G	FAT: 9 G	PROTEIN: 18 G

INGREDIENTS

- handful of pitted olives
- ¼ tsp pepper
- 2 large eggs
- 3 tbsp feta cheese, crumbled
- ½ scallion, chopped thinly
- 1 tsp olive oil
- ½ bell pepper, chopped thinly

DIRECTIONS

1. In a mixing bowl, whisk the eggs before adding the bell pepper, cheese, black pepper, olives, and scallions.
2. Pour the egg mixture into a pan over medium heat with olive oil. Allow the mixture to cook for about 2 minutes then start scrambling it.
3. Continue to stir for 3 minutes or until the eggs are cooked through.
4. Enjoy this dish hot.

Gluten-Free Muffins

Cinnamon is a scent associated with warmth and baking, and now you can enjoy it in a muffin. With crunchy almonds, sweet carrots, and currents, with just a hint of cinnamon, these oats-based treats will become your new favorite snack. Enjoy fresh from the oven or with some of your favorite preserves.

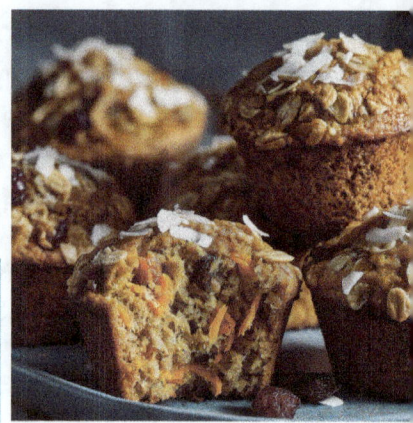

TIME: 50 MIN	SERVINGS: 12 (24 mini muffins)	PREP: 30 MIN	COOK: 20 MIN
CALORIES: 159 KCAL	CARBS: 24.6 G	FAT: 6.2 G	PROTEIN: 3.1 G

INGREDIENTS

- 1 tbsp unsweetened shredded coconut, garnish
- ¼ tsp baking soda
- 1½ cups rolled oats, gluten-free
- 1 cup unsweetened applesauce
- 1 cup carrot, shredded and coarsely chopped
- ⅔ cup light brown sugar
- 1 tsp ground cinnamon
- 2 large eggs
- ⅓ cup almonds, chopped
- 2 tbsp olive oil
- 1 tsp baking powder
- ¼ tsp salt
- ⅓ cup currants
- 1 tsp vanilla extra

DIRECTIONS

1. Preheat the oven to 350 °F.
2. Prepare a 24-cup mini muffin tin with some olive oil.
3. Add the oats to a blender and blend until finely ground before adding the baking powder, cinnamon, baking soda, and salt, then pulse a couple of times.
4. Pour in the apple sauce, eggs, oil, vanilla, and brown sugar, then blend until smooth.
5. Add the nuts, currents, and carrots, then stir.
6. Pour the mixture into the prepared muffin tin and top with the shredded coconut.
7. Bake the muffins for no more than 20 minutes. Use a toothpick to ensure the muffin is baked all the way through.
8. Remove the muffins from the baking tin, and allow them to cool on a wire rack for 10 minutes.
9. Eat them once cool, or freeze them for later enjoyment.

Shrimp Zoodles

Shrimp brings a salty-sweet blend of flavors that are enhanced by salty olives and sweet tomatoes. While tasty on their own, the shrimp are best enjoyed with zoodles and some Greek seasoning to bring the whole dish together. Enjoy the shrimp hot or allow them to cool before adding them to uncooked zoodles and other toppings.

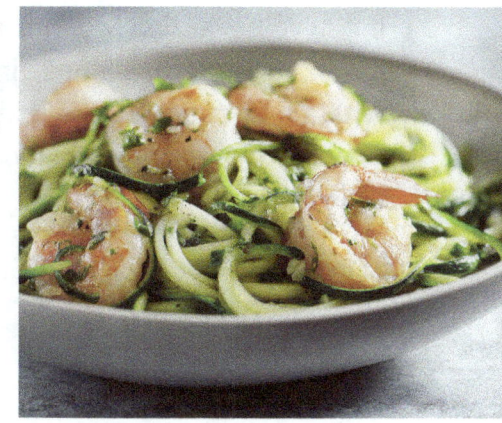

TIME: 20 MIN	SERVINGS: 2	PREP: 10 MIN	COOK: 10 MIN
CALORIES: 621 KCAL	CARBS: 16 G	FAT: 48 G	PROTEIN: 35 G

INGREDIENTS

FOR SHRIMP:
- 8 oz large shrimp, peeled and deveined
- 2 large zucchinis, spiralized (directions in the Chicken and Zoodles with Pesto recipe)
- ¼ tsp pepper
- 2 tbsp virgin olive oil
- ¼ tsp salt
- 1 tsp Greek seasoning

TOPPINGS INGREDIENTS:
- ½ cup kalamata olives, pitted
- 2 tbsp virgin olive oil
- ½ pint cherry tomatoes
- ½ tbsp red wine vinegar
- ½ tsp salt
- 1 tsp Greek seasoning
- 4 oz feta cheese dairy-free (optional)

DIRECTIONS

1. In a large skillet, add 2 tablespoons of oil and raise the temperature to medium.
2. Add all the shrimp ingredients—excluding the zoodles—and cook the shrimp for 2–3 minutes a side or until cooked through.
3. Place the zoodles in the skillet and toss them together with the shrimp.
4. Add the topping ingredients to the zoodle mixture and cook for another 1–2 minutes before serving hot.

Moroccan Chicken Stew

If you've never had Moroccan chicken stew, this hearty meal makes a regular chicken meal look tired. This stew is full of herbs and spices, with a hint of sweetness that can make any dreary rainy day into one of warmth and comfort. Enjoy over some quinoa or gluten-free bread.

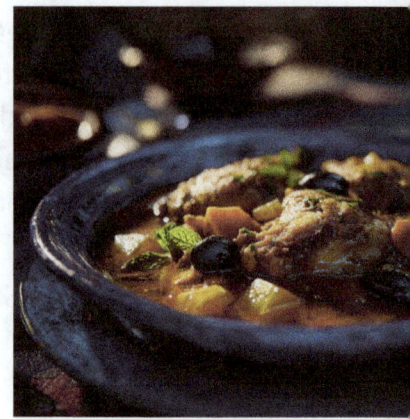

TIME: 27 MIN	SERVINGS: 4	PREP: 5 MIN	COOK: 22 MIN
CALORIES: 304 KCAL	CARBS: 41.9 G	FAT: 8.6 G	PROTEIN: 14.9 G

INGREDIENTS

- 3 cups chicken broth, divided
- ¼ tsp salt
- 1 tbsp olive oil
- ½ cup black olives
- 1 tbsp fresh mint
- ¼ cup lemon juice
- 1 lb chicken thighs, skinless
- 1 tsp chili powder
- 1 cup quinoa
- 1 cup onion, diced
- 1 cup of carrot, peeled and diced

DIRECTIONS

1. Add some olive oil to a pan and cook the chicken for 2–3 minutes a side. Remove the meat and cover to keep warm.
2. Add all the spices to the pan and toast for a few minutes before adding the onion and carrots. Cook until the carrots soften and the onions start to turn clear.
3. Pour in 2 cups of chicken broth, lemon juice, and olives before bringing the mixture to a boil over high heat.
4. Return the chicken to the mixture and cover the pan, and then allow the mixture to simmer for 10–15 minutes.
5. While the chicken is simmering, prepare the quinoa with a cup of chicken broth. Boil the broth in a saucepan before adding the quinoa. Remove the saucepan from the heat before covering it, allowing it to stand for at least 10 minutes.
6. Fluff the quinoa after it's cooked before gently stirring in the mint leaves.
7. Once the chicken is cooked, season to taste.
8. Split the quinoa between 4 bowls before topping it with chicken and ½ cup of the sauce.
9. Add chili to taste before serving.

IDEAS TO ELEVATE THIS MOROCCAN CHICKEN STEW:

- Serve it with a sprinkle of fresh mint or a dollop of yogurt for a cooling contrast to the spices.
- Add ½ to 1 teaspoon of harissa paste or a pinch of cayenne pepper to the stew while sautéing the onions. Harissa, a North African chili paste, will infuse the dish with a smoky, spicy kick that complements the Moroccan flavors beautifully.
- Pair it with a side of warm, toasted pita bread or a light cucumber salad to round out the meal.

Grilled Salmon Salad

This grilled salmon salad is perfect for someone who doesn't have time to marinate a piece of fish but still expects all the flavors as if it were. The subtly seasoned salmon with its yogurt dressing is perfect for any summertime feast, especially when accompanied by a fresh, crunchy salad bursting with color and taste.

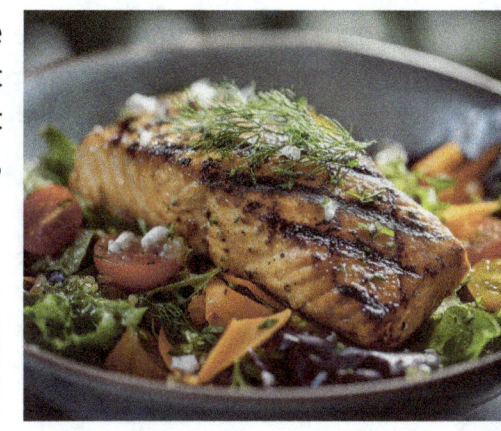

TIME: 30 MIN	SERVINGS: 6	PREP: 15 MIN	COOK: 15 MIN
CALORIES: 242 KCAL	CARBS: 7 G	FAT: 12 G	PROTEIN: 25 G

INGREDIENTS

FOR SALMON:
- 1 ½ lb salmon filet
- ¼ tsp salt
- ¼ tsp pepper

FOR DRESSING:
- ⅛ tsp salt
- ½ cup Greek yogurt
- ¼ tsp black pepper
- 2 tsp honey
- 1 tbsp Dijon mustard
- ¼ cup chopped fresh dill
- 2 tbsp olive oil
- 2 tbsp freshly squeezed lemon juice

FOR SALAD:
- 2 cups mesclun salad mix
- 2 radishes, sliced thin
- 1 cucumber, peeled and sliced
- ¼ red onion, sliced into thin rings
- 2 carrots, grated
- fresh parsley, garnish
- fresh oregano, garnish

DIRECTIONS

1. Preheat the oven to grill.
2. Lay the fish on a baking tray and season both sides with salt and pepper. Set aside.
3. In a small bowl, whisk all the salad dressing ingredients.
4. In a large bowl, add all the salad ingredients and toss.
5. Place the fish in the oven, and cook for about 5 minutes before flipping and cooking for a few more minutes on the other side. This may be longer or shorter depending on the thickness of the fish.
6. Add the fish to the salad before pouring the dressing over and serving immediately with the preferred garnish. Alternatively, allow the fish to cool before adding it to the salad.

Polenta Pizza

Thanks to polenta, you can enjoy a gluten-free pizza without resorting to a gluten-free base. The recipe below only contains a smidgen of toppings you can enjoy, so experiment to see which best suits your tastes.

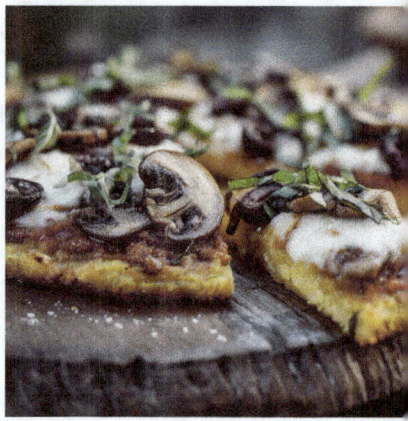

TIME: 1 Hr	SERVINGS: 6	PREP: 10 MIN	COOK: 50 MIN
CALORIES: 409 KCAL	CARBS: 31 G	FAT: 28 G	PROTEIN: 10 G

INGREDIENTS

FOR POLENTA CRUST:
- 1 cup instant polenta (cooks quicker)
- 1 tsp salt
- 1 cup milk or milk alternative
- ¼ cups olive oil
- 3 cups water

FOR MUSHROOM AND ONION TOPPING:
- 10 oz mushrooms, sliced
- 1 tsp dried thyme
- 2 onions, halved and sliced thin
- ¼ cup red wine
- ¼ cup olive oil

FOR REMAINING TOPPINGS:
- ½ cup tomato sauce
- 1 cup kalamata olives, pitted
- 1 cup mozzarella, shredded

DIRECTIONS

1. Preheat the oven to 400 °F.
2. Add oil to a pizza pan or a cookie sheet and set aside.
3. In a saucepan, pour in the water, milk, a teaspoon of salt, and ¼ cup of olive oil before bringing the mixture to a boil.
4. Slowly stir in the polenta to avoid lumps forming. Lower the heat and stir the polenta mixture for about 5 minutes until it thickens. Remove the saucepan from the heat.
5. Pour the polenta onto the prepared pan or sheet and press it down to the desired pizza thickness.
6. Bake the polenta pizza base for 35 minutes.
7. As the crust bakes, add the mushrooms, onions, and ¼ cup olive oil in a pan for 3 minutes before adding the thyme, wine, and ¼ teaspoon salt. Allow the mixture to cook for 3–5 minutes, allowing most of the liquid to cook away. Remove the sauce from the heat.
8. Move the pizza from the oven and coat it with the tomato sauce before adding the onion and mushroom mixture.
9. Top the pizza with olives and cheese and continue to bake the pizza for another 15 minutes.
10. Serve hot or cold.

Quinoa and Kale Stew

The quinoa and kale stew aren't only filling; it complements well with red lentils, making this stew a winner at any dinner table. Quinoa and kale are both superfoods that are packed with nutrients, and adding red lentils to the mix adds even more protein and fiber.

TIME: 40 MIN	SERVINGS: 4	PREP: 15 MIN	COOK: 35 MIN
CALORIES: 367 KCAL	CARBS: 61.9 G	FAT: 5.9 G	PROTEIN: 19.1 G

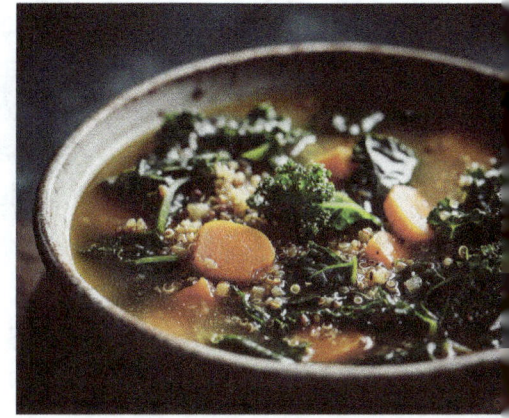

INGREDIENTS

- ½ tsp ground turmeric
- 4 clove garlic, minced
- ½ cup quinoa
- ½ tsp ground ginger
- 1 tbsp coconut oil
- 3 celery stalks
- 1 cup red lentils
- 1 ½ tsp ground cumin
- 26.5 oz tomatoes, diced
- 1 onion, chopped
- 5 cup water
- 1 ½ tsp ground cumin
- 2 tsp salt
- 3 carrot, chopped
- 2 cup kale, chopped

DIRECTIONS

1. Melt the coconut oil in a large pot over medium heat before adding the celery, carrots, and onion to sauté for 8 minutes until soft.
2. Add the garlic and cook until fragrant.
3. Pour in the water, tomatoes, ginger, lentils, cumin, salt, quinoa, and turmeric, and then bring the mixture to a boil.
4. Lower the heat to bring it to a simmer. Keep it there for about 20 minutes or until all the vegetables are soft.
5. Add the kale and cook long enough for the leaves to start wilting.
6. Split the meal between 4 bowls and serve immediately. Season as desired.

Caprese Pasta Salad

There is nothing more Mediterranean than a Caprese salad. To give a unique twist to an old classic, add some slivers of olive and fresh basil to breathe new life into it. Combine with rich mozzarella, sweet tomatoes, and gluten-free pasta and you'll have a light meal or several sides at a family dinner. Enjoy as fresh as possible to get the unique blend of flavors.

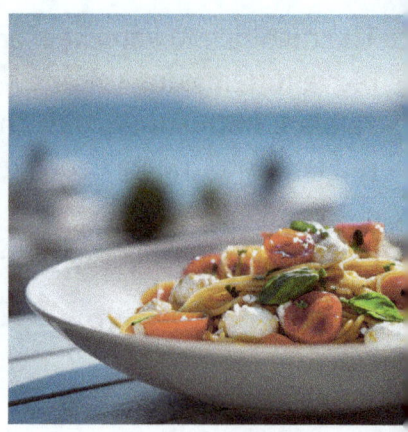

TIME: 16 MIN	SERVINGS: 4	PREP: 10 MIN	COOK: 6 MIN
CALORIES: 363 KCAL	CARBS: 49.1 G	FAT: 12.1 G	PROTEIN: 13.4 G

INGREDIENTS

- ¼ cup fresh basil, rinsed, dried, and cut into ⅛-inch wide silvers
- 8 oz gluten-free spaghetti
- 8 black olives, pitted and cut into slivers
- 1 tbsp olive oil
- 3 oz mozzarella cheese, cubed
- 4 tomato rinsed, cored and cubed

DIRECTIONS

1. Add 3 quarts of water to a large pot and bring to a boil.
2. Follow the instructions on cooking your preferred gluten-free pasta brand.
3. Once the pasta is cooked, remove a cup of water and set it aside before draining the rest.
4. Return the pasta to the pot before adding the olive oil and enough reserved water to coat the pasta.
5. Then add the olives, tomatoes, mozzarella, and basil, then toss and serve.

Turkey Skillet Meal

In as little as 30 minutes, the flavors of tomato, oregano, and garlic will be wafting from a skillet full of ground turkey. While the tomato gives a slight citrus tang to the dish the basil and zucchini cut through the sourness with their mild sweetness. Truly a meal for anyone pressed for time.

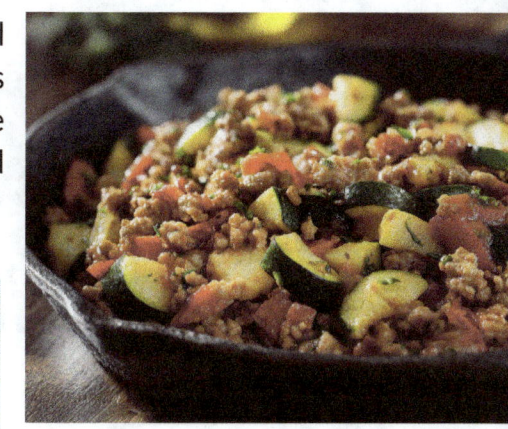

TIME: 40 MIN	SERVINGS: 4	PREP: 15 MIN	COOK: 25 MIN
CALORIES: 223 KCAL	CARBS: 12.5 G	FAT: 9.8 G	PROTEIN: 26.3 G

INGREDIENTS

- ¾ lb ground turkey
- 2 zucchini, chopped in quarter rounds or zoodles (directions in Chicken and Zoodles with Pesto recipe)
- 1 onion, chopped
- ¼ ground black pepper
- 3 tomatoes, chopped
- ½ tsp salt
- 3 tbsp tomato paste
- 1 tsp garlic powder
- 1 tp ground oregano
- 1 tsp dried basil

DIRECTIONS

1. Lightly coat a large skillet with some olive oil.
2. Add the ground turkey and onion, and cook the mixture over medium heat until the onions are soft and the turkey is cooked; roughly 10 minutes.
3. To this mixture, pour in the herbs, spices, tomato paste, and tomatoes. Lower the heat to medium and let the mixture simmer for 10 minutes.
4. Place the chopped zucchini in the pot, mix well, and continue to cook for 5 minutes before serving hot

IDEAS TO ELEVATE THIS TURKEY SKILLET MEAL:

- To make the Turkey Skillet Meal spicy and elevate its flavor, add ½ teaspoon of crushed red pepper flakes or a dash of chili oil when sautéing the garlic and turkey.
- This will introduce a subtle heat that balances beautifully with the sweetness of the basil and zucchini, creating a more dynamic and flavorful dish. For an extra boost, garnish with a drizzle of spicy harissa oil or a sprinkle of freshly chopped chili before serving.

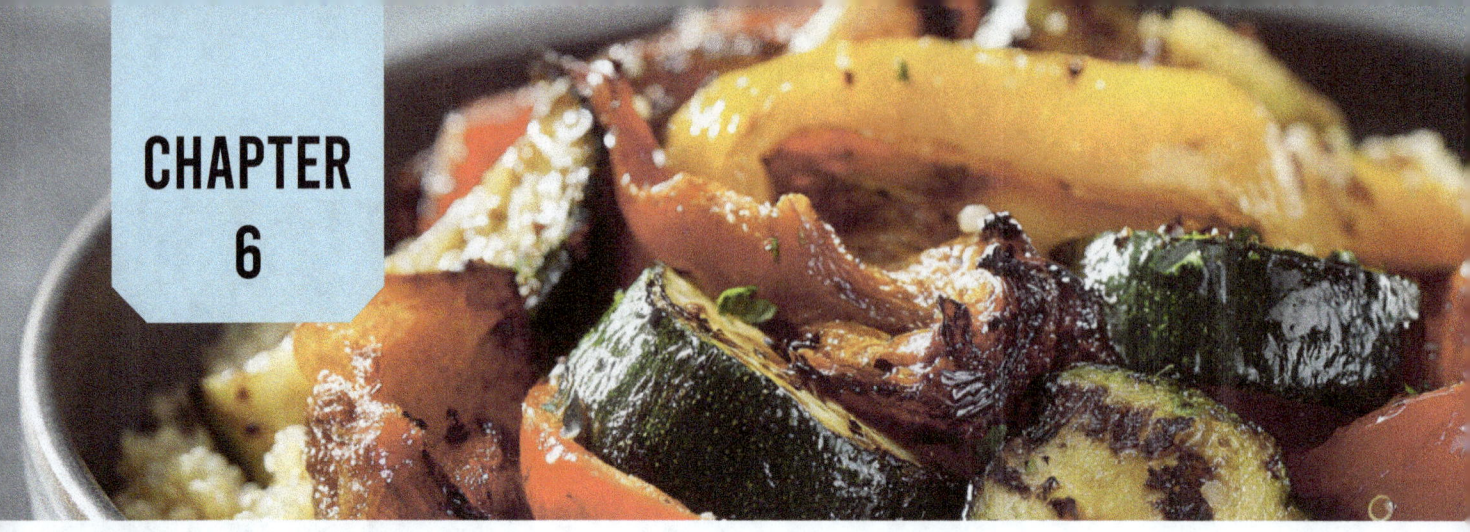

CHAPTER 6

Vegan-Friendly
MEDITERRANEAN

The Mediterranean diet is celebrated for its vibrant, fresh, and wholesome ingredients, making it a natural fit for vegan-friendly adaptations. A vegan diet excludes all animal products, including meat, dairy, eggs, and even honey, embracing a plant-based lifestyle that prioritizes health, environmental sustainability, and compassion for animals.

In the Mediterranean culinary tradition, many staples align beautifully with vegan principles. Fresh vegetables like eggplant, zucchini, and bell peppers, nutrient-rich legumes like chickpeas and lentils, and whole grains like bulgur and farro take center stage.

Healthy fats from olive oil and a medley of herbs such as basil, oregano, and rosemary add depth and flavor, creating dishes that are as nutritious as they are delicious.

This chapter explores how traditional Mediterranean foods can be transformed into vegan delights while preserving their signature flavors. Recipes emphasize whole, fiber-rich ingredients, which not only aid in weight management but also support heart health and stabilize blood sugar levels.

Complex carbohydrates like whole grains and legumes provide slow-digesting energy, helping to prevent blood sugar spikes and improve insulin sensitivity. Additionally, the absence of cholesterol in a vegan diet—found only in animal products—makes these recipes especially heart-friendly.

From hearty vegetable stews to creamy hummus and vibrant salads, these vegan Mediterranean dishes will bring the taste of the sun-soaked coasts to your table. Whether you're exploring veganism for health, ethics, or environmental reasons, this chapter is your gateway to enjoying the best of Mediterranean cuisine without compromise.

Meal Planning and Preparation

While it's easy to say "avoid animal products," it's not as easy for some as it seems to others. It may be easy to avoid seafood (fish, crustaceans, and shellfish), meat, dairy, and eggs, but it's difficult to avoid all animal-based ingredients unless you know what you're looking for.

Some hidden animal-based ingredients include whey, casein, gelatin, and omega-3 fatty acids, and those are just a few. This isn't the only hurdle a vegan eater has to get across.

Due to the restrictiveness of this diet, deficiencies may occur if your diet is poorly planned. Some of the more common deficiencies experienced include

- vitamin B12
- vitamin D
- long-chain omega-3 fatty acids
- iodine
- iron
- calcium
- zinc (Petre, 2022)

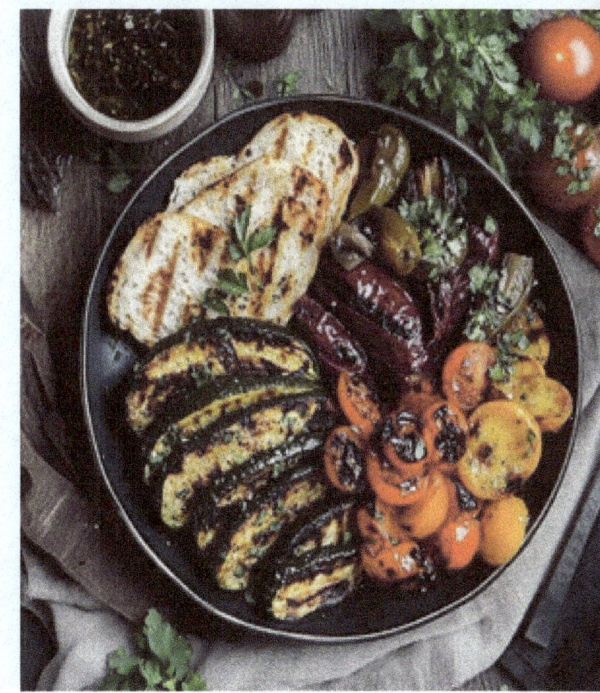

These deficiencies will become more apparent in those who do a lot of training or may be pregnant. However, with enough planning, a vegan diet doesn't have to have these deficiencies. Iodine can easily be added to a diet by eating seaweed and using iodized salt.

Iodine is vital as it isn't needed to make thyroid hormones. Long-chain omega-3 fatty acids—such as eicosapentaenoic and docosahexaenoic acid (EPA and DHA)—can be made by the body through the consumption of alpha-linolenic acid (ALA) (Petre, 2022). Foods high in ALA include chia, flaxseeds, soybeans, walnuts, and hemp.

Another deficiency noted is the lack of protein. While plant-based proteins may not be as readily available as animal-based proteins, many different plant-based foods give the required protein needed for an optimal lifestyle. It all comes down to planning, preparing, and getting your shopping list together.

Becoming a vegan after enjoying the life of an omnivore can be a drastic step and requires some preparation before diving into it. Start by becoming a flexitarian—someone who switches out animal-based meals for plant-based meals—before becoming vegetarian and finally becoming a vegan. However, if you're comfortable making the full switch, then, by all means, do.

Vegans will benefit from the Mediterranean diet since it does not require specific grains, fruits, vegetables, nuts, seeds, or legumes. Nevertheless, dairy, eggs, and meat are all no-goes when a vegan diet is followed. So, you'll need to update your shopping list to eat safely on a Mediterranean diet.

Food Types	Examples
Dairy substitutes	✓ Plant-based milk (almond, rice, hemp, coconut, oats, and cashew; depending on taste and preference), plant-based cheeses (almond, coconut, and cashew), and yogurt made with coconut, almond, or cashew. » Consider brands such as Daiya, Almond Breeze, or Go Veggie. » Should be fortified with calcium and vitamins B12 and D.
Egg substitutes	✓ Vegan eggs are easy to make with either chia seeds or ground flaxseeds. » Made with 3 tablespoons of warm water. » These seeds are high in protein and omega-3 fatty acids. » Used to replace eggs in quiches or frittatas. ✓ Scrambled tofu and mashed banana can be used, depending on the recipe.
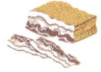 Protein	✓ All legumes enjoyed with the Mediterranean diet. » Try combinations of raw, cooked, fermented, or even sprouted. ✓ While not strictly from the Mediterranean region, tofu, seitan, and tempeh can replace meat. ✓ Algae (spirulina and chlorella) has protein and iodine. ✓ Nutritional yeast helps with a cheesy flavor and can be fortified with vitamin B12.
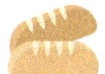 Fermented and sprouted	✓ Other foods you can try include: Ezekiel bread (whole grains and sprouted legumes), miso, natto, sauerkraut, pickles, kimchi, and kombucha. ✓ These foods provide not only protein but help with strengthening gut biomes (Petre, 2022).

While there are no limitations on fruit and vegetables, it's a good idea to concentrate on dark green, leafy vegetables. Vegetables such as bok choy, spinach, watercress, and mustard greens are high in iron and provide much-needed calcium.

Broccoli and Tofu

Tofu can take on the taste of anything you add to it. With a mixture of honey, ginger, soy sauce, and sesame oil, the tofu will take on a tangy-sweet flavor, perfect for crispy, sautéed broccoli. Combine with couscous, rice, or quinoa for a filling meal.

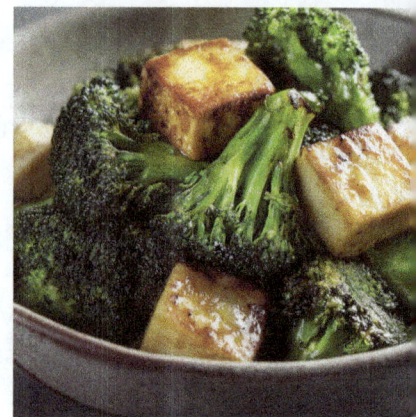

TIME: 21 MIN	SERVINGS: 4	PREP: 10 MIN	COOK: 11 MIN
CALORIES: 190 KCAL	CARBS: 13.9 G	FAT: 1.9 G	PROTEIN: 13.8 G

INGREDIENTS

- 1 lb broccoli florets
- 1 tbsp peanut oil
- 16 oz tofu firm, drained
- 1 tbsp fresh ginger, chopped finely
- 2 tbsp soy sauce
- ½ tbsp honey
- 8 clove garlic, minced
- ¼ tsp red pepper flakes
- 1 tsp sesame oil
- 1 tbsp sesame seeds (optional)

DIRECTIONS

1. Cut the tofu into 8 pieces and place them on a flat plate on top of 4 paper towels. Add 4 towels on top and place a cutting board over that. Gently press down to squeeze the moisture out. Continue to add dry towel paper and press down until no more liquid is released. This will help the tofu absorb more flavor.
2. Add the dried tofu to a large bowl and lay the pieces so they don't overlap.
3. Create the marinade by pouring the soy sauce, ginger, sesame oil, and honey into a small bowl and whisk well until the honey is dissolved. Pour the liquid over the tofu before turning the pieces to coat them well. Set aside.
4. Add some olive oil to a sauté pan before adding the broccoli and cooking for 5 minutes. Remove the vegetables from the pan.
5. Raise the temperature to high, add the drained tofu—keeping the marinade—and grill for 3 minutes. Turn the cooked side up and grill the tofu for another 3 minutes.
6. While the tofu is done cooking, lower the temperature to medium-low and add the peanut oil with the garlic and red pepper. Cook for no more than a minute before adding the broccoli and the leftover marinade.
7. Gently stir until everything in the pan is well-coated.
8. Serve with a sprinkle of some sesame seeds.

Vegan-Friendly Pilaf

While the cherries bring a tang of sweetness to the pilaf, the pine nuts and the quinoa bring their own earthy undertone. The combination of flavors and textures will make everyone want a bite of your meal. The pilaf can last several days in the fridge.

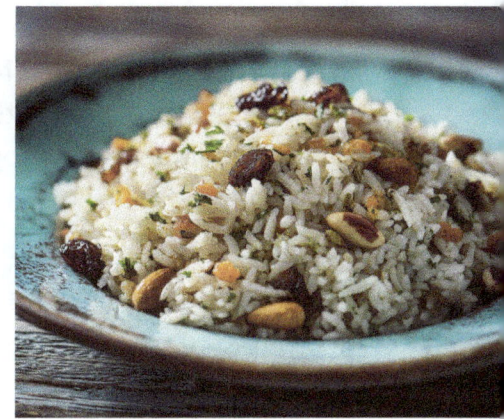

TIME: 30 MIN	SERVINGS: 4	PREP: 8 MIN	COOK: 22 MIN
CALORIES: 81 KCAL	CARBS: 13.7 G	FAT: 2 G	PROTEIN: 2.2 G

INGREDIENTS

- ½ cup fresh parsley
- 1 tsp salt
- ½ cup cherries, dried
- 1 tsp ground black pepper
- ¼ cup pine nuts
- 1 clove garlic, minced
- 2 cups vegetable broth
- 1 cup red quinoa, rinsed

DIRECTIONS

1. Add the broth to a saucepan and boil over medium-high heat.
2. Pour in the quinoa and garlic before stirring.
3. Lower the temperature until the mixture starts to simmer, and cook for 12–15 minutes. Most of the liquid should be absorbed during this time.
4. Add the cherries, stir, cover, and allow the mixture to cook for another 7 minutes.
5. During this time, add the pine nuts to a smaller pan and roast them for a few minutes.
6. Serve the pilaf with a sprinkle of roasted pine nuts.

Mediterranean Hummus Bowl

Hummus is a standard dip used in most Mediterranean snacks or mezze platters. It's a go-to for people as a snack with vegetables. To create a meal, combine nutty quinoa with a rainbow of colors with spinach, cucumbers, tomatoes, onions, and olives. Group the various colors together to make a visually pleasing and tasty meal.

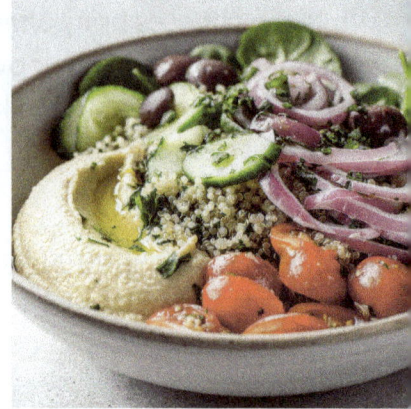

TIME: 15 MIN	SERVINGS: 4	PREP: 15 MIN	COOK: None
CALORIES: 324 KCAL	CARBS: 44 G	FAT: 12 G	PROTEIN: 14 G

INGREDIENTS

FOR THE HUMMUS:
- 2–3 ice cubes
- 15 oz canned chickpeas
- ½ tsp salt
- 3 tbsp lemon juice
- 1–2 garlic cloves
- 2 tbsp tahini (recipe found in Lettuce Wraps with Tahini Dressing)

FOR THE BOWL:
- 1 cup canned chickpeas, skins removed
- ½ pint cherry tomatoes, quartered
- 1 cup cooked quinoa
- ½ English cucumbers, sliced
- ½ cup olives, pitted
- ½ red onion, sliced
- 2 cups baby spinach
- parsley, chopped, for serving
- olive oil, for serving

DIRECTIONS

1. Add the chickpeas to a food processor and blend them until they become powder-like.
2. Place the ice cubes, tahini, salt, lemon juice, and garlic cloves in the food processor and blend until smooth. Season with salt or lemon to taste.
3. Scrape out the hummus and place it in a large bowl before topping it with the various bowl ingredients before serving.

Burbara

Burbara is a wheat berry pudding full of spice, nuts, and dried fruit that can be served hot or cold. Often eaten as a dessert, burbara is a creamy pudding that incorporates all the flavors of the Middle East. While traditionally made with wheat berries, these can be difficult to find in most grocery stores. By using pearled barley, the creaminess is retained, and a pleasant chewiness remains.

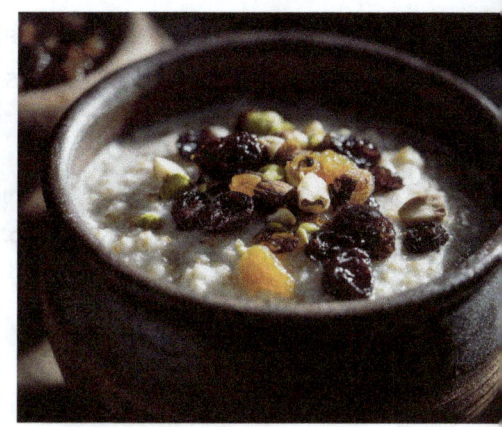

TIME: 45 MIN	SERVINGS: 6	PREP: 5 MIN	COOK: 40 MIN
CALORIES: 212.1 KCAL	CARBS: 50.5 G	FAT: 0.6 G	PROTEIN: 4.1 G

INGREDIENTS

- 1 cup pearled barley
- ½ cup dried cherries
- 1 tsp ground cinnamon
- ½ cup dried apricots, chopped with
- extra for garnish
- 4 tbsp honey
- ½ tsp fennel seeds
- 1 tsp anise seeds
- nuts of choice for garnish, use almonds, walnuts, or pistachios
- pomegranate seeds, garnish

DIRECTIONS

1. Add 4 cups of water to your barley in a saucepan and boil over medium-high heat. Once a boil is reached, lower the heat to bring the mixture to a simmer for 20 minutes, then cover. Be sure to stir now and again to prevent the barley from sticking.

2. Once cooked, remove the lid and add the fennel seeds, cinnamon, anise seeds, dried fruit, and honey. Stir to mix well, and cook for 15–20 minutes. Stir and check occasionally and stop cooking once the barley is fully cooked. A sure sign that the dish is ready is that the fruit becomes plump, and the mixture becomes creamy.

3. Serve the dessert garnished with pomegranate seeds, dried fruit, and nuts. Alternatively, allow to cool and refrigerate for later before garnishing.

Green Olive Salad with Pomegranate Molasses

Not everyone is fond of the unique tangy-tart taste of green olives. However, this recipe comes together with a splash of pomegranate molasses dressing that cuts through the tartness.

TIME: 10 MIN	SERVINGS: 2	PREP: 10 MIN	COOK: None
CALORIES: 213 KCAL	CARBS: 21.3 G	FAT: 14.7 G	PROTEIN: 2.6 G

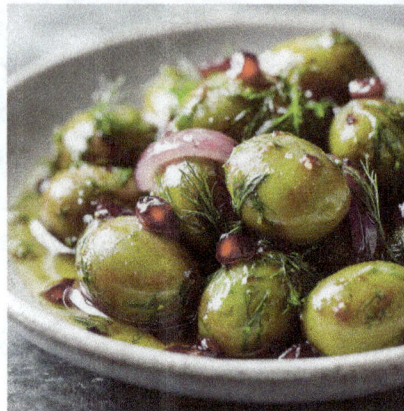

INGREDIENTS

FOR DRESSING:
- 1 tbsp lemon juice
- 1 tbsp pomegranate molasses
- 2 tbsp olive oil

FOR SALAD:
- 1 red onion, chopped
- 1 cup green olives, pitted
- ¼ tsp salt
- ¼ cup fresh dill, chopped
- 1 tsp sumac
- ¼ cup parsley, chopped
- 1 cup grape tomatoes, halved
- 1 green onion, chopped (optional)

DIRECTIONS

1. Add the salt, onion, and sumac to a medium bowl, and stir until the onion is well coated.
2. Add the remaining herbs with the tomatoes and green onions and toss the salad. Set aside.
3. In a small bowl, pour the olive oil, lemon juice, and pomegranate molasses, then whisk well.
4. Immediately pour the dressing over the salad and stir to coat everything before serving.

Lettuce Wraps with Tahini Dressing

Lettuce wraps are a great quick and easy meal that can be placed in a lunch box or enjoyed immediately. The flavor of the tahini brings a nutty, almost earthy, flavor to the bean-like taste of the chickpeas. With the addition of toasted almonds, it won't only be the lettuce that brings a crisp crunch to this meal.

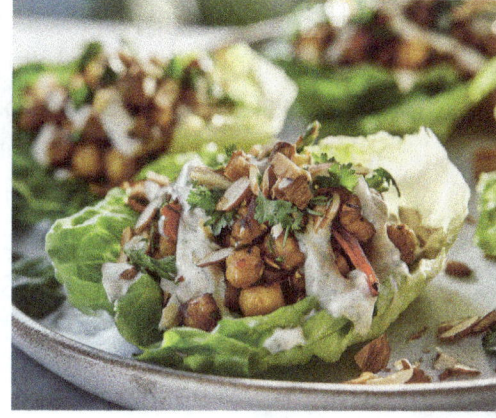

TIME: 17 MIN	SERVINGS: 4 (12 Wraps)	PREP: 12 MIN	COOK: 5 MIN
CALORIES: 498 KCAL	CARBS: 43.7 G	FAT: 28 G	PROTEIN: 15.8 G

INGREDIENTS

FOR TAHINI:
- 3 tbsp olive oil
- 4 cups hulled sesame seeds

FOR WRAPS:
- 2 (15 oz) cans chickpeas, rinsed
- 12 large Bibb lettuce leaves (or other large, pliable lettuce)
- ¾ tsp kosher salt
- ¼ cup tahini
- 2 tbsp chopped fresh parsley
- ¼ cup olive oil
- ¼ cup toasted almonds, chopped
- 1 tsp lemon zest
- ½ cup shallots, sliced thinly
- ¼ cup lemon juice
- ½ cup jarred roasted red peppers, drained and sliced
- 1 ½ tsp pure maple syrup
- ½ tsp paprika

DIRECTIONS

FOR TAHINI
1. Add the sesame seeds to a skillet and cook over medium-low until they turn slightly golden; roughly 5 minutes.
2. Allow the seeds to cool to room temperature, add to a blender and blend for a minute on high until a paste forms.
3. Pour in the olive oil and blend for 1 minute until the paste becomes creamy.
4. Once complete, add the tahini to a sealable container and keep it in your fridge until it's needed.

FOR WRAPS:
1. In a bowl, whisk the paprika, oil, tahini, salt, maple syrup, lemon juice, and zest before adding the shallots, chickpeas, and peppers. Stir the ingredients until well-coated.
2. Scoop ⅓ cup of the contents onto the lettuce leaves before topping with parsley and almonds before wrapping tightly.

Vegetable and Bean Salad with Basil Vinaigrette

Salads should never be bland or boring; if they are, then you aren't adding enough flavors. With fresh and juicy vegetables accompanied by a basil vinaigrette, the combination of flavors is straight out of the Mediterranean. Even the cannellini beans bring their own nutty taste to help enhance the other flavors waiting to be discovered.

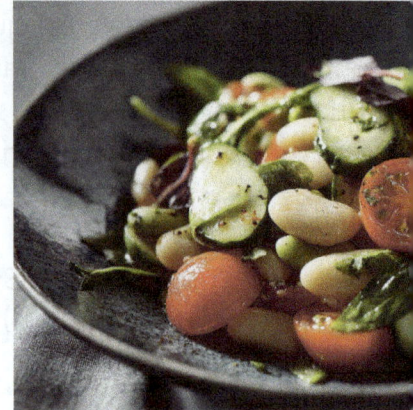

TIME: 25 MIN	SERVINGS: 4	PREP: 25 MIN	COOK: None
CALORIES: 246 KCAL	CARBS: 21.5 G	FAT: 15.3 G	PROTEIN: 7.5 G

INGREDIENTS

- 1 cup halved cherry tomatoes
- 3 tbsp red-wine vinegar
- 1 (15 oz) can cannellini beans, rinsed
- ½ cup fresh basil leaves, packed (slightly squashed into measuring tool)
- 1 tbsp finely chopped shallot
- ½ cucumber (~ 1 cup), halved lengthwise and sliced
- 2 tsp Dijon mustard
- ¼ tsp salt
- ¼ cup olive oil
- 1 tsp honey
- ¼ tsp ground pepper
- 10 cups mixed salad greens

DIRECTIONS

1. Add the greens, beans, cucumber, and tomatoes to a large salad bowl and set aside.
2. To make the basil vinaigrette, add the salt, pepper, basil, honey, oil, mustard, vinegar, and shallot to a food processor and blend until the mixture is smooth.
3. Pour over the salad and enjoy immediately.

Roasted Vegetable Bowl

Roast vegetables give a beautiful smoky taste to the underwhelming flavor of the chickpeas. Meanwhile, the red pesto wraps the meal up with its tangy sweetness. With the beautiful colors from the roasted bell peppers, onion, and broccoli, you'll soon be enjoying a rainbow feast.

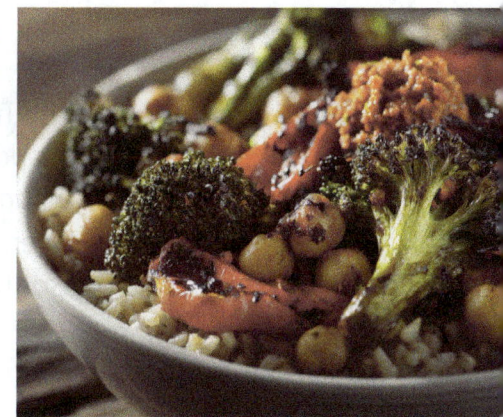

TIME: 35 MIN	SERVINGS: 4	PREP: 15 MIN	COOK: 20 MIN
CALORIES: 484 KCAL	CARBS: 64.4 G	FAT: 20.5 G	PROTEIN: 12.4 G

INGREDIENTS

- 1 (15 oz) can chickpeas, rinsed
- 3 cups cooked brown rice
- ½ tsp garlic powder
- ¼ tsp salt
- ¼ tsp ground pepper
- 2 medium red bell peppers, quartered
- 4 tbsp red pesto (recipe found in Mediterranean Gnocchi)
- 4 cups broccoli florets
- 1 cup red onion, sliced
- 3 tbsp virgin olive oil, divided

DIRECTIONS

1. Preheat the oven to 450 °F.
2. In a large bowl, add the salt, pepper, garlic powder, and 2 tablespoons of oil before whisking.
3. Add the onion, peppers, and broccoli before tossing them.
4. Lay the coated vegetables on a rimmed baking sheet in a single layer before placing them in the oven to roast for 20 minutes.
5. Pour the remaining oil into the cooked rice and stir well before dividing into 4 bowls.
6. Split the roast vegetables and chickpeas between the containers before topping the mixture with a tablespoon of pesto.
7. Serve hot or cold. If reheating, add the food to a microwave-safe container and heat it for 1–2 minutes on high.

Roasted Red Pepper Hummus with Quinoa Chickpea Salad

Roasted red peppers are known for their smoky sweetness, which makes them an excellent addition to hummus. This uniquely flavored hummus goes hand in hand with the nuttiness of the quinoa. Add some sunflower seeds to enhance the nuttiness and crunch. You can even roast them before sprinkling them over the dish.

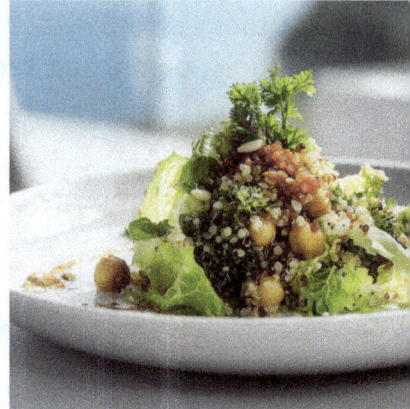

TIME: 15 MIN	SERVINGS: 1 (~ 3 ½ cups)	PREP: 15 MIN	COOK: None
CALORIES: 379 KCAL	CARBS: 58.5 G	FAT: 10.5 G	PROTEIN: 16 G

INGREDIENTS

- 1 tbsp sunflower seeds, unsalted
- 2 tbsp hummus (recipe from the Mediterranean Hummus Bowl recipe)
- ½ cup cooked quinoa
- a pinch of ground pepper
- ½ cup chickpeas, rinsed
- 1 tbsp
- lemon juice
- a pinch of salt
- 2 cups mixed salad greens
- 1 tbsp roasted red pepper, chopped
- 1 tbsp fresh parsley, chopped

DIRECTIONS

1. In a small dish, add the hummus, red peppers, and lemon juice before stirring until well combined. If the mixture is too thick, add some water to thin to a dressing consistency. Add a teaspoon at a time to prevent making it too thin.
2. In another bowl, add the chickpeas, greens, and quinoa before topping the bowl with salt, pepper, sunflower seeds, and parsley.
3. Drizzle the dressing over then enjoy.

Mediterranean Vegan Pasta

A combination of walnuts and hummus creates a creamy pasta sauce that's almost good enough to eat as is. While olives give their saltiness to the dish, it's the optional cranberries that bring a tart sweetness and color. Serve the fragrant sauce while the pasta is hot and enjoy the scents wafting from your dinner plate.

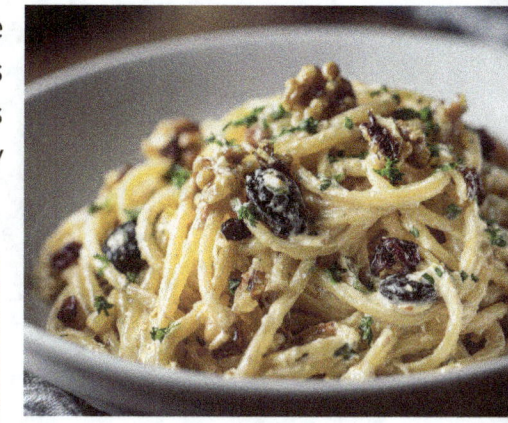

TIME: 15 MIN	SERVINGS: 6 (12 cups)	PREP: 5 MIN	COOK: 10 MIN
CALORIES: 620 KCAL	CARBS: 79 G	FAT: 12 G	PROTEIN: 26 G

INGREDIENTS

- 10 oz preferred pasta
- ½ cup walnuts
- 1 cup hummus (from the Mediterranean Hummus Bowl recipe)
- 5 cloves garlic, minced
- ⅓ cup water
- ½ cup olives
- ¼ tsp pepper
- ¼ tsp salt
- 2 tbsp dried cranberries (optional)

DIRECTIONS

1. Cook pasta as instructed by the manufacturer's directions.
2. As the pasta is cooking, make the hummus sauce. In a bowl, mix the garlic, hummus, and water before seasoning to taste.
3. Add the walnuts, dried cranberries, and olives.
4. Once the pasta is cooked, drain it well and serve it with the sauce.

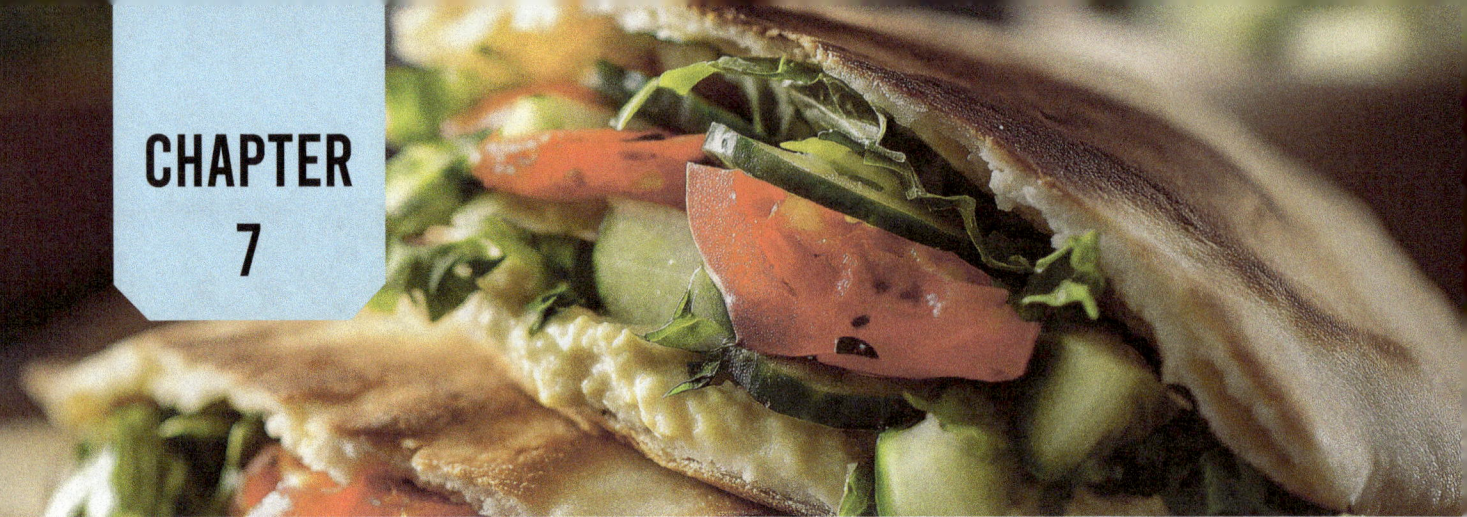

CHAPTER 7

Vegetarian-Friendly MEDITERRANEAN

The vegetarian diet is more forgiving in what you can eat than the vegan diet. People on a vegetarian diet only refrain from eating any meat and animal by-products such as gelatin. Other animal products, such as dairy and eggs, are often enjoyed depending on the type of vegetarian, as some refrain from eating one or the other.

Similar to the vegan diet, if a vegetarian diet isn't well planned, it results in deficiencies in vitamin B12, iron, calcium (not consuming dairy), and zinc, which are more readily absorbed from meat than plants (Baker, 2021). Luckily, with proper planning, the impact of these deficiencies can be minimized.

Vitamin B12 can be found in fortified cereals, milk, and eggs. Iron can be absorbed by enjoying dried fruits and beans, tofu, and lentils. For people who are ovo-vegetarians (only consume eggs but not milk), they will need to increase how much green leafy vegetables, such as broccoli and okra, they eat, and drink fortified milk alternatives. Zinc is abundant in nuts, seeds, mushrooms, and even wheat germ.

Because the Mediterranean diet leans toward eating more plant-based than animal-based meals, it goes hand in hand with living a vegetarian lifestyle. Most meals eaten throughout the Mediterranean are vegetarian-friendly or can easily be adapted.

While it may seem difficult to plan a well-balanced vegetarian diet, don't give up hope. There are many resources available to you. Nutiro can help with its random food generator and meal plans.

Meal Planning and Preparation

Fruits and vegetables will take up most of your diet, and because of this, concentrate on the shelf life of what you're purchasing. You don't need to stick to fresh—which usually only lasts a week in some cases—so make use of dried, frozen, or canned varieties. Be sure that most of the recipes you use contain ingredients you enjoy eating, not just eating them because they're vegetarian-friendly.

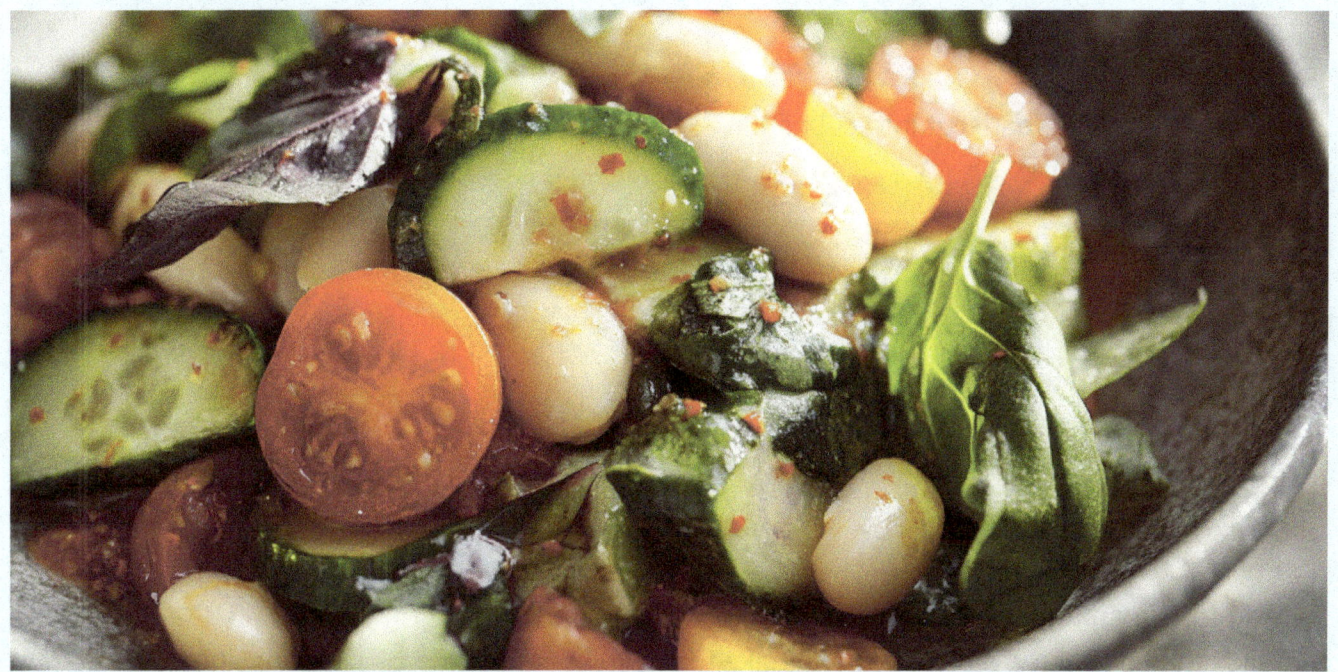

Switching from an omnivore to a vegetarian is significantly easier than switching to a vegan lifestyle. Start by excluding meat-based dishes a few times a week, and replace them with plant-based meals.

The Mediterranean way of eating leans more toward a plant-based lifestyle, so if you're already a vegetarian, there are minuscule changes you'll need to make. As a vegetarian, don't eat meat, poultry, and seafood. Everything else you can enjoy.

To prevent deficiencies in this diet, consider on adding these foods to your Mediterranean diet.
- Protein and Iron: Legumes, seitan, tempeh, lentils, and chickpeas
- B12: Dairy, eggs, fortified cereals, and nutritional yeast

Mozzarella Omelet

The mixture of mozzarella, tomato, and basil brings an otherwise flavorless scrambled egg white to life with flavor. Never before has a plain breakfast been so tasty and unique. Especially after adding the homemade croutons that are folded into the eggs to give a pleasant crunch.

TIME: 35 MIN	SERVINGS: 1	PREP: 10 MIN	COOK: 25 MIN
CALORIES: 320 KCAL	CARBS: 19.9 G	FAT: 10 G	PROTEIN: 32.2 G

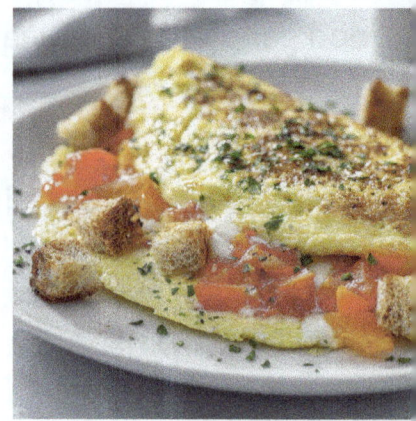

INGREDIENTS

- ½ slice artisan bread, cut into cubes
- 1 tsp dried basil
- ½ tsp olive oil
- 1 tomato, chopped
- 1 clove garlic, chopped finely
- 2 tbsp mozzarella cheese, grated
- ¾ cup egg whites

DIRECTIONS

1. Preheat the oven to 300 °F.
2. Add the bread to a small bowl and toss with oil and garlic.
3. Place the cubes on a baking tray and bake for 15 minutes or until desired crispiness. Toss a few times to bake equally. Set aside to cool.
4. Coat a skillet with olive oil and raise the temperature to medium-high before adding the eggs.
5. Spread the egg out in the skillet and allow it to set before lowering the temperature.
6. Allow the eggs to cook until the top is almost cooked before scattering the basil, tomato, cheese, and bread cubes over half of the egg. Gently fold the other half over this and cook covered for a few more minutes.
7. Slide the omelet onto a plate and serve hot.

Lemon Ricotta Pancakes

Pancakes are a sweet start to any morning, and this recipe is no exception. The ricotta makes a fluffy pancake, while the lemon and maple syrup flavors battle it out between tangy and sweet.

TIME: 30 MIN	SERVINGS: 4 (~ 8 pancakes)	PREP: 10 MIN	COOK: 50 MIN
CALORIES: 281 KCAL	CARBS: 34 G	FAT: 10 G	PROTEIN: 13 G

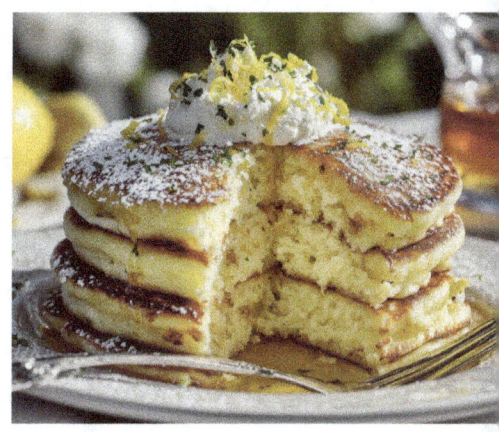

INGREDIENTS

- 1 tbsp olive oil
- 1 tbsp lemon juice
- ½ cup all-purpose flour
- ½ cup buttermilk
- 2 tbsp granulated sugar
- 2 large eggs
- ½ cup whole-grain flour
- ¾ cup ricotta cheese
- 1 tsp vanilla extract
- ⅛ tsp salt
- 1½ tsp baking powder
- maple syrup, for serving
- 2 tsp grated lemon zest, plus more for garnish

DIRECTIONS

1. Sift the dry ingredients into a large bowl.
2. In a separate bowl, whisk the lemon components, ricotta, vanilla, buttermilk, oil, and eggs until smooth before pouring it into the dry ingredients. Mix well.
3. Over medium heat, add a skillet lightly coated with some oil.
4. Once hot, pour ¼ cup of batter per pancake into the pan and cook until bubbles begin to form and the edges are dry. Flip and cook the other side for another 2-3 minutes. Reduce heat if the pancakes brown too quickly.
5. Serve hot pancakes with some lemon zest and a drizzle of maple syrup.

Mediterranean Grill Tofu

With herbs and spices from every corner of the Mediterranean, it's hard to find something more flavorful to snack on. The tofu is a sponge for this rich flavor and holds up well during grilling. There will always be leftover marinade sauce that can be served along with fresh pita or Greek salad shared in the Stuffed Avocados recipe.

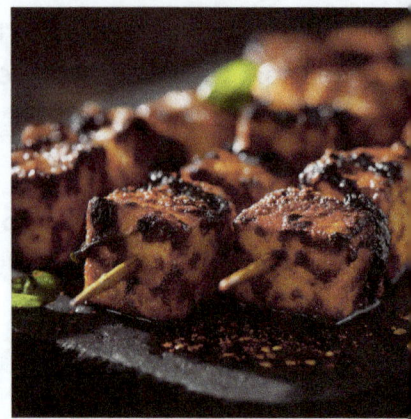

TIME: 1 Hr	SERVINGS: 2	PREP: 45 MIN	COOK: 15 MIN
CALORIES: 605 KCAL	CARBS: 12.6 G	FAT: 54.8 G	PROTEIN: 20.9 G

INGREDIENTS

- ½ tsp cumin
- ¼ tsp cayenne
- 1 package (14 oz) extra firm tofu
- ½ tsp turmeric
- 1 tbsp tomato paste
- ½ tsp onion powder
- 1 tsp honey
- ¼ tsp coriander
- 2 tbsp lemon juice
- ½ tsp garlic powder
- 1 tsp dried oregano
- ¼ tsp cinnamon
- ⅓ cup olive oil
- ½ tsp paprika
- ¾ tsp salt

DIRECTIONS

1. Drain the tofu before wrapping it in a paper towel and applying a heavy item to it. Set aside for 30 minutes to pull moisture from the tofu.
2. Heat the grill to medium.
3. Add the remaining ingredients to a small bowl and whisk until a paste forms.
4. Cut the tofu into cubes, thread them into some skewers, and apply the marinade. Don't throw away any excess marinade.
5. Allow the tofu cubes to rest for 15 minutes before adding them to the grill.
6. Cook 3–5 minutes a side, only allowing a slight char before rotating. Apply some excess marinade while grilling for extra flavoring. Serve hot.

Greek Yogurt Parfait

Yogurt parfaits are a layered treat combining creamy Greek yogurt, fresh fruits, and crunchy granola or nuts. They're a versatile and healthy option, perfect for breakfast, snacks, or dessert, offering a balance of flavors and textures in every bite.

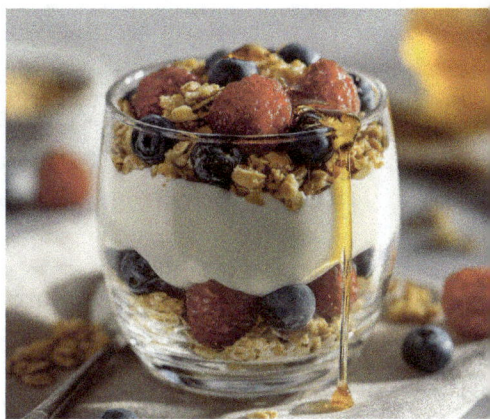

TIME: 10 MIN	SERVINGS: 8 (8 Cups)	PREP: 10 MIN	COOK: None
CALORIES: 232 KCAL	CARBS: 27.7 G	FAT: 10.3 G	PROTEIN: 8.3 G

INGREDIENTS

- 1 ½–2 cups of granola
- 1 (32 oz) container of Greek yogurt
- 1 lb of fresh or frozen berries or fruit
- 3 tbsp honey (optional)

DIRECTIONS

1. Gather 1½–2 cups of granola, 32 oz of Greek yogurt, 1 lb of fresh or frozen berries or fruit, and 3 tbsp honey if using.
2. In serving glasses or bowls, layer the ingredients:
    a. Start with a spoonful of Greek yogurt at the bottom.
    b. Add a layer of granola.
    c. Follow with a layer of berries or fruit.
    d. Repeat the layers until the glass or bowl is full.
3. Drizzle honey on top for added sweetness, if desired.

Orecchiette with Broccoli and Basil Sauce

If you're having trouble eating all your greens, look no further than a generous helping of delicious ear-shaped pasta filled with creamy, vibrant green sauce. While the zucchini and broccoli give their slightly bitter-sweet taste to the dish, it's the parmesan that creates the creamy aftertaste that brings the dish together.

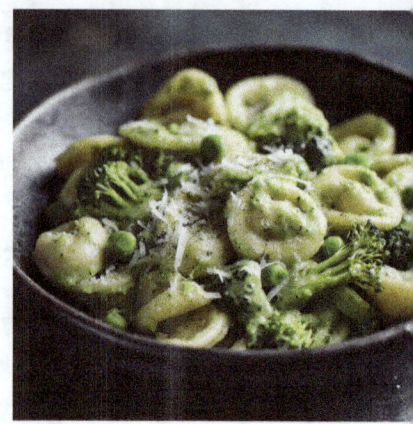

TIME: 30 MIN	SERVINGS: 4	PREP: 10 MIN	COOK: 20 MIN
CALORIES: 498 KCAL	CARBS: 66.7 G	FAT: 17.7 G	PROTEIN: 20.3 G

INGREDIENTS

- 7 oz broccoli florets
- 8.8 oz orecchiette
- 1 zucchini, chopped
- 2 cups peas
- 1 clove garlic, peeled
- 1 cup fresh basil
- 5.3 oz cream cheese
- 1 pinch ground black pepper
- 2 tbsp parmesan cheese, grated
- 1 tbsp parmesan cheese, garnish

DIRECTIONS

1. In a large saucepan, add the garlic, broccoli, zucchini, and enough water to cover them. Boil for 5 minutes before removing the vegetables and retain the water.
2. Add the vegetables to a blender with ½ cup of the cooking water, pepper, parmesan, basil, and cream cheese before blending until smooth.
3. Cook the pasta in the vegetable water until al dente. Drain well.
4. In a clean saucepan, add the broccoli sauce and the peas before cooking them over low temperature for 2–3 minutes.
5. Add in the pasta and stir before dishing. Serve with some parmesan and pepper.

Lentil Salad

Cooked lentils have a delightfully nutty and peppery taste, which goes hand in hand with just about anything. Toss in some fresh cherry tomatoes, crunchy cucumbers, and salty olives, and you have a dish made in heaven. This meal will last up to 5 days in the fridge if you don't eat it all in one sitting.

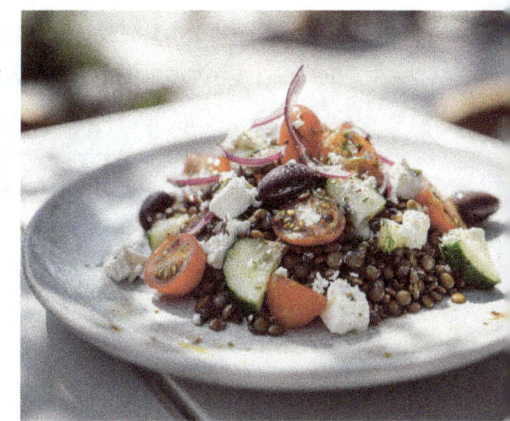

TIME: 10 MIN	SERVINGS: 6	PREP: 7 MIN	COOK: None
CALORIES: 271 KCAL	CARBS: 25 G	FAT: 15 G	PROTEIN: 11 G

INGREDIENTS

- ½ tsp ground pepper, divided
- 3 cups cooked brown lentils
- ½ cup feta cheese, crumbled
- ¼ cup olive oil
- 3 tbsp red wine vinegar
- 1 pint cherry tomatoes, halved
- ½ cup red onion, thinly sliced
- ½ tsp honey
- 1 tbsp shallot, chopped finely
- 1 ½ cups cucumber, chopped
- ½ cup kalamata olives, pitted and coarsely chopped
- ½ tsp garlic, minced
- ½ tsp salt, divided

DIRECTIONS

1. In a large bowl, add ¼ teaspoon of salt and pepper, the lentils, feta, tomatoes, onion, cucumber, and olives before combining.
2. In a separate bowl, whisk the remaining salt and pepper, vinegar, honey, shallot, and garlic. Pour in the oil while whisking the ingredients.
3. Drizzle the oil mixture over the lentil mixture and toss before serving.

Greek Salad with Hummus

This is a light and tasty lunch inspired by the classic Greek salad. Add some extra avocado if you want to make it even more filling.

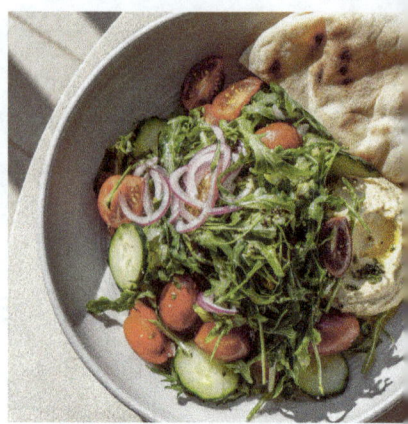

TIME: 10 MIN	SERVINGS: 1	PREP: 10 MIN	COOK: None
CALORIES: 422 KCAL	CARBS: 30.5 G	FAT: 29.9 G	PROTEIN: 10.9 G

INGREDIENTS

- 2 tsp red-wine vinegar
- 2 cups arugula
- ⅛ tsp ground pepper
- ¼ cup hummus (recipe from the Mediterranean Hummus Bowl recipe)
- 1 ½ tbsp olive oil
- ⅓ cup cherry tomatoes, halved
- 1 tbsp red onion, chopped
- 1 (4-inch) whole-wheat pita
- 1 tbsp feta cheese
- ⅓ cup cucumber, sliced

DIRECTIONS

1. Whisk red wine vinegar, olive oil, and pepper in a small bowl.
2. Toss arugula, tomatoes, cucumber, and red onion with the dressing.
3. Toast the pita and cut into wedges.
4. Spread hummus on a plate, top with salad, and sprinkle with feta.
5. Serve with pita and optional avocado. Enjoy!

Veggie Wrap with Cilantro Hummus

There are many ways to make hummus, each way not only unique in color but also in taste. This cilantro hummus is sure to make your veggie wrap pop with flavor, and it lasts 3 days in the fridge.

TIME: 20 MIN	SERVINGS: 4	PREP: 20 MIN	COOK: None
CALORIES: 269 KCAL	CARBS: 35.1 G	FAT: 12.1 G	PROTEIN: 15.6 G

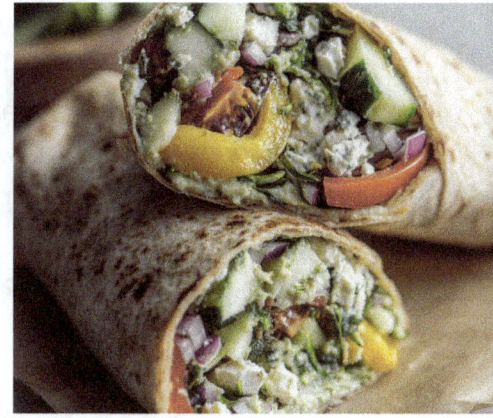

INGREDIENTS

FOR THE HUMMUS:
- 1 (15 oz) can chickpeas, rinsed
- 2 tbsp olive oil
- ¼ cup fresh cilantro leaves
- 1 tbsp tahini (found in the Lettuce Wraps with Tahini Dressing recipe)
- 1 clove garlic, peeled and minced
- 3 tbsp lemon juice
- ¼ tsp white pepper
- ¼ tsp salt

FOR THE WRAP:
- 2 tbsp bottled mild banana peppers (or pepperoncini), sliced
- 4 (8-inch) multi-grain wraps
- 1 tbsp balsamic vinegar
- ½ large cucumber, halved lengthwise and sliced
- ¼ cup feta cheese, crumbled
- ¼ tsp black pepper
- 1 tbsp olive oil
- 1 cup chopped tomato
- ½ cup thinly sliced red onion
- 1 clove garlic, minced
- 4 cups mixed baby green

DIRECTIONS

1. Add all the hummus ingredients—excluding the cilantro—to a blender and blend until smooth.
2. Add the fresh cilantro and pulse a few times to distribute the herb. Scoop the hummus from the blender and set aside.
3. In a large bowl, add the greens, banana peppers, cucumber, feta cheese, tomato, and red onion, and mix.
4. Make the dressing in a smaller bowl by whisking the black pepper, vinegar, garlic, and olive oil before drizzling it over the salad. Toss well.
5. Lay the wraps out and spread 2 ½ tablespoons of hummus before topping with the greens mixture.
6. Roll tightly and serve immediately.

Mediterranean Quiche

With a baked base filled with egg, sweet spinach, tart sun-dried tomatoes, and olives, just having one bite will make you feel that you're enjoying the quiche at a cafe in the Mediterranean. Being light and savory, the quiche goes well with potatoes, Greek salad (from the Stuffed Avocados recipe), or can be enjoyed as is.

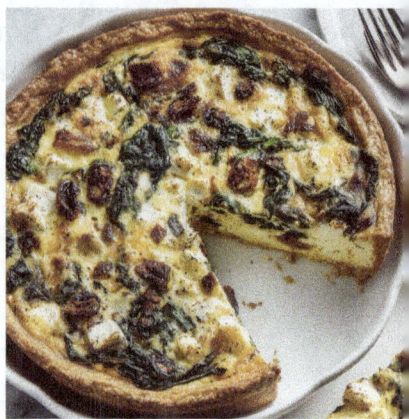

TIME: 55 MIN	SERVINGS: 6 (~ 6 slices)	PREP: 10 MIN	COOK: 45 MIN
CALORIES: 195 KCAL	CARBS: 4.7 G	FAT: 15.1 G	PROTEIN: 10.8 G

INGREDIENTS

FOR THE CRUST:
- 3 tsp fresh basil, chopped
- ⅛ tsp ground black pepper
- 2 tsp olive oil
- ½ tsp garlic powder
- 2 cups almond flour
- ½ tsp kosher salt
- 1 large egg

FOR THE FILLING:
- 5 large eggs
- 2 cups spinach, packed (slightly squashed into measuring tool)
- 1 cup almond milk, unsweetened
- ½ cup feta cubes
- ⅓ cup kalamata olives, pitted
- ⅓ cup sun-dried tomatoes
- ¼ tsp pepper

DIRECTIONS

1. Preheat the oven to 400 °F and prepare a 10-inch pie plate with olive oil.
2. In a bowl, add all the dry ingredients for the crust and stir until combined. Pour in the oil and eggs, then use a fork to incorporate them with the dry ingredients.
3. Press the crumbly dough into the prepared pan along the bottom and sides before baking it for 15–20 minutes. The edges of the crust should start to brown.
4. Remove the crust from the oven and layer the olives, spinach, and sun-dried tomatoes.
5. In a clean bowl, add the remaining fillings ingredients and whisk well before pouring them over the vegetables.
6. Return the pie plate to the oven and cook for another 30–35 minutes. The filling should be set before serving.

Baked Feta Pasta

There is nothing more beautiful than the blood red of the tomatoes as it surrounds the white of the feta. One swirl of a spoon helps blend these colors together to create the creamy sauce that will accompany pasta. Don't forget to add fresh spinach and basil to bring their unique sweetness to the salty dish.

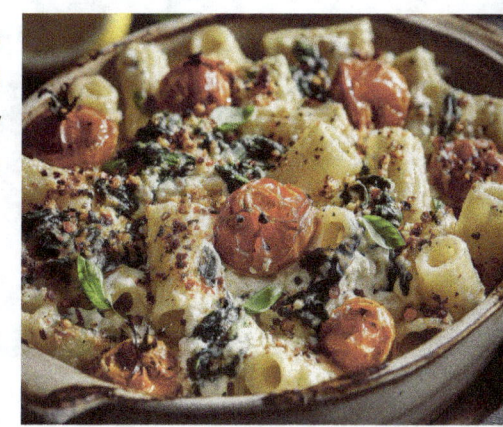

TIME: 40 MIN	SERVINGS: 4	PREP: 5 MIN	COOK: 35 MIN
CALORIES: 380 KCAL	CARBS: 31 G	FAT: 8 G	PROTEIN: 5 G

INGREDIENTS

- handful fresh basil, chopped and extra for serving
- 1 (16 oz) package of cherry tomatoes
- 2-3 tbsp olive oil
- 2 cups cooked pasta
- 1 (7 oz) block of feta
- handful of baby spinach
- ¼ tsp pepper
- 1 tsp dried Italian seasoning
- ¼ tsp salt
- 2-3 garlic cloves, minced and divided

OPTIONAL INGREDIENTS:
- dried herbs such as rosemary, oregano, or basil
- red pepper chili flakes
- lemon zest or lemon juice

DIRECTIONS

1. Preheat the oven to 400 °F.
2. Place the tomatoes in a casserole dish and then add the seasoning, salt, pepper, olive oil, and half the garlic.
3. Create a well in the center and place the feta. Season with dried oregano and bake for 30–35 minutes. The tomatoes should start bursting open.
4. Prepare the pasta while the feta is baking and drain it well.
5. After the feta is baked, add half the basil before stirring the mixture until a creamy texture is reached.
6. Tip in the pasta, remaining garlic, and spinach, and toss gently to coat well.
7. Season and add the remaining basil before serving hot.

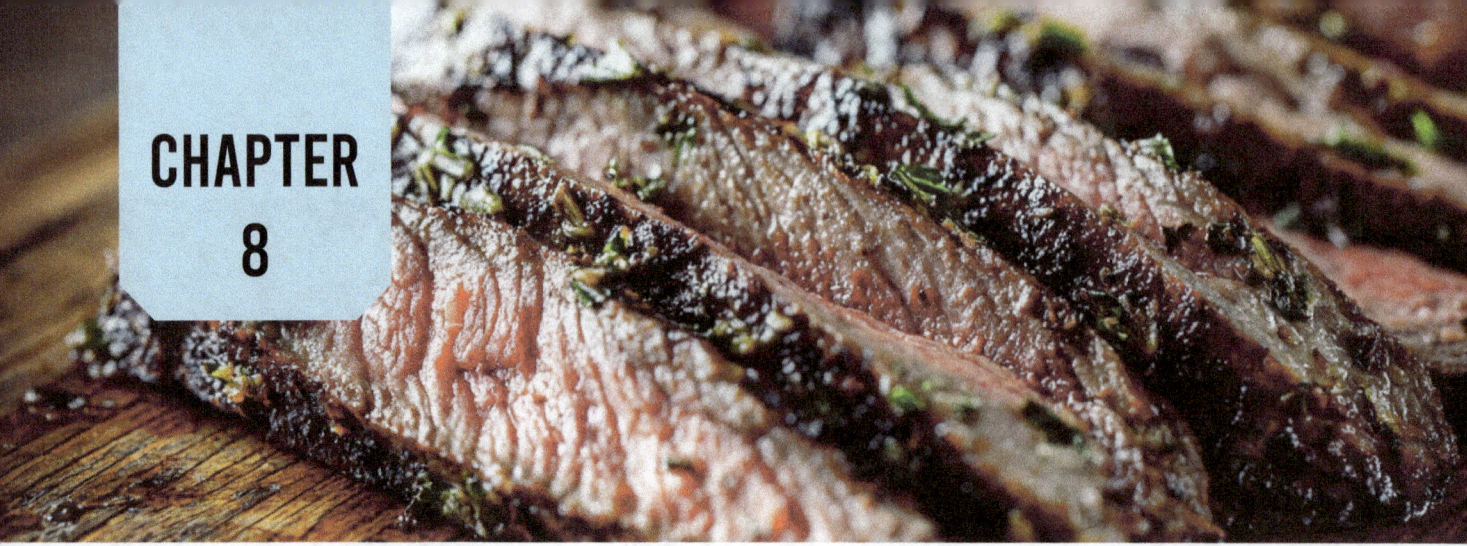

CHAPTER 8

Paleo-Friendly MEDITERRANEAN

The idea behind the paleo diet is that human eating habits should return to the way of our hunter-gatherer ancestors. Before agriculture and the domestication of what would become farm animals. The diet consists of eating lean meats, seafood, fruits, vegetables, nuts, and seeds while shunning dairy, grains, and all processed foods. In some cases, even legumes aren't eaten.

One of the biggest concerns on this diet is getting enough fiber and calcium. The deficiency can, however, be compensated for by eating plenty of fruits and vegetables. You can even include psyllium husk to aid in digestion.

Whole foods are encouraged on the paleo diet, but many condiments aren't allowed because they contain gluten. Meat and vegetable stocks need to be prepared at home, rather than purchased, to prevent accidentally consuming gluten. Making your own stocks means you can also make bone broth.

Meal Planning and Preparation

You may have to look at the ingredients of your favorite recipes to determine if they are paleo-friendly. Many recipes on the internet may say they are paleo-friendly but then contain butter or ghee. Strictly speaking, no dairy products are allowed on paleo. However, some people use gluten-free grains and grass-fed butter, even though this isn't strictly paleo-friendly.

In terms of the Mediterranean diet, you will need to remove all grains, dairy products, and legumes if you want to be a strict paleo eater. For calcium and fiber, you'll need to consume dark green, leafy vegetables.

You will also need to avoid overly processed foods, so concentrate on how your healthy oils are made. Coconut oil should be as unrefined as possible, so look for phrases such as organic virgin coconut oil. Alternatively, use olive oil.

As with previously mentioned meals, preparing a paleo meal plan comes down to what you want to eat. Some ingredients last longer than others in the fridge and need to be stored frozen or canned instead. When buying canned goods, read the label to ensure the food hasn't been overly processed, as you want to eat as much whole food as possible.

Zesty Mediterranean Chicken Salad

A tangy apple cider vinegar dressing smothering chicken is the perfect go-to lunch. Combine that with crunchy carrots and cabbage alongside some fiery ginger, and you have a plate bursting with color. Skip the cilantro if it's not to your taste.

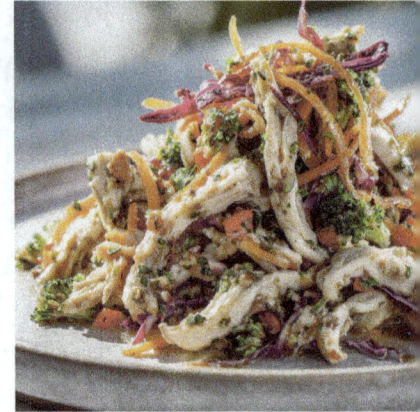

TIME: 10 MIN	SERVINGS: 4	PREP: 10 MIN	COOK: None
CALORIES: 318 KCAL	CARBS: 16 G	FAT: 18.4 G	PROTEIN: 23.3 G

INGREDIENTS

- 1 ½ cup broccoli
- ¼ cup minced ginger
- ¼ cup cilantro, chopped
- 3 cooked chicken breasts, cut into strips
- ¼ cup orange juice
- carrots, cleaned and cut into strips
- 2 cups red cabbage, shredded
- 3 green onions, sliced
- ½ cup salad dressing, ¼ cup apple cider vinegar, and ¼ olive oil
- 1 red bell pepper, cut into strips

DIRECTIONS

1. In a small bowl, add the homemade salad dressing, lemon juice, and ginger and whisk.
2. Add the chicken to a medium bowl with the cabbage, onion, bell pepper, broccoli, and carrots before drizzling the salad dressing over.
3. Gently stir in the cilantro and serve.

Paleo-Mediterranean Frittata

A frittata is so much more than just an egg-based dish. Bursting with the rich flavors from the artichokes, tomatoes, and olives, you'll find that it fills all the requirements of a filling meal. This frittata combines the nutrient-dense ingredients and bold flavors typical of the Mediterranean diet while adhering to Paleo principles by avoiding grains, dairy, and processed foods.

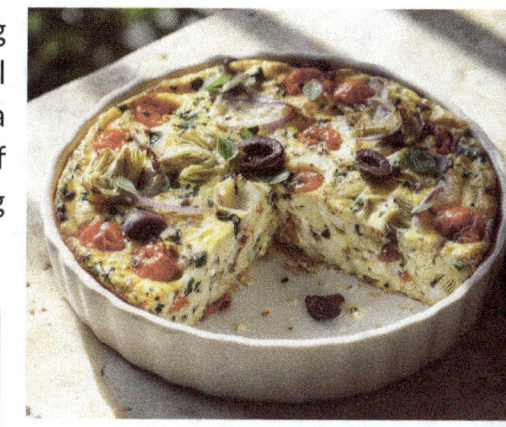

TIME: 1 Hr	SERVINGS: 8	PREP: 20 MIN	COOK: 40 MIN
CALORIES: 256 KCAL	CARBS: 6 G	FAT: 20 G	PROTEIN: 11 G

INGREDIENTS

- 12 eggs
- ½ cup fresh basil, sliced
- ½ red onion, diced
- 1 (14.5 oz) can artichoke hearts, drained and quartered
- 2 cups grape or cherry tomatoes, halved
- ¼ cup coconut milk
- ¼ tsp salt
- 1 cup kalamata olives, sliced
- ¼ tsp pepper
- 2 cups spinach, roughly chopped
- 2 tbsp coconut oil

DIRECTIONS

1. Preheat the oven to 375 °F.
2. Prepare a baking dish with some olive oil and set aside.
3. In a separate bowl, add the eggs and coconut milk before whisking.
4. Add all the chopped vegetables to the egg mixture, season to taste, and then mix.
5. Add this mixture to the baking dish and bake for 40–45 minutes, or until the center of the dish is cooked through. Start checking doneness from about 30 minutes into baking time.
6. Once done, serve hot, or allow to cool before refrigerating.

Zesty Lemon Bars

Indulge your sweet tooth with a combination of tangy lemon and sweet maple syrup. Before you know it, everyone will want a little bite of your lemony treats. Chilling the bars will ensure a clean cut when serving.

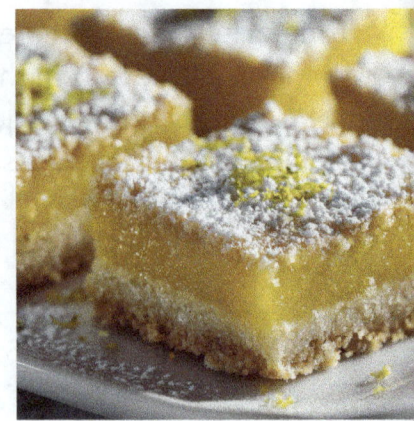

TIME: 4 Hr 50 MIN	SERVINGS: 12 (12 Bars)	PREP: 10 MIN + 4 Hr Chilling	COOK: 40 MIN
CALORIES: 189 KCAL	CARBS: 18.9 G	FAT: 11.5 G	PROTEIN: 4.9 G

INGREDIENTS

FOR CRUST:
- 1 ½ cups fine blanched almond flour, packed (slightly squashed into measuring tool)
- ¼ tsp salt
- ¼ tsp almond extract
- ¼ cup pure maple syrup
- 2 tbsp coconut flour
- ¼ cup coconut oil, melted

FOR FILLING:
- zest from 1 lemon, extra for garnish
- 1 tbsp coconut flour
- ⅔ cup lemon juice
- 4 large eggs
- ½ cup pure maple syrup

DIRECTIONS

1. Preheat the oven to 350 °F.
2. Add some parchment paper to an 8 x 8-inch pan, and set aside.
3. In a bowl, stir the salt and the flour together. Then add the almond extract, coconut oil, and maple syrup before mixing to form a dough.
4. Press the dough into the prepared pan and bake for 15 minutes.
5. While the dough bakes, in a fresh bowl, add the coconut flour, lemon zest, eggs, lemon juice, and maple syrup before whisking until no more egg white is visible.
6. After the crust is done but still hot, pour the filling in.
7. Lower the oven to 325 °F, place the pan back into the oven and bake for 20–25 minutes until the filling is set.
8. Allow the pan to cool down then add to the fridge for 4 hours.
9. When ready to serve, cut into 12 bars, and scatter lemon zest over the top.

Apple Tuna Bites

While grains are an important part of the Mediterranean diet, so are a variety of fruit. Swap bread for the sweet tang of a fresh apple, accompanied by a healthy serving of tuna for a delicious snack.

TIME: 15 MIN	SERVINGS: 1	PREP: 15 MIN	COOK: None
CALORIES: 377 KCAL	CARBS: 26 G	FAT: 11 G	PROTEIN: 42 G

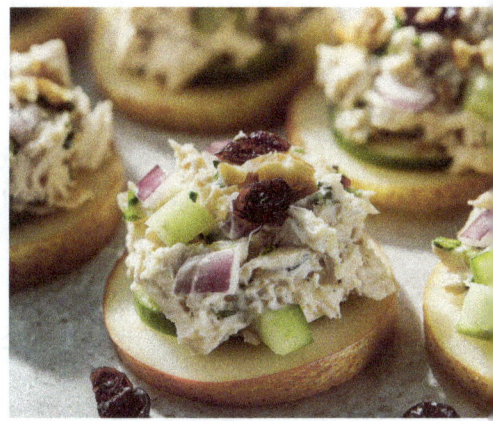

INGREDIENTS

- 2 tbsp coconut yogurt
- ¼ tsp pepper
- 5 oz tuna, drained
- 1 tsp fresh lemon juice
- 2 tbsp red onion, diced
- ¼ cup celery, chopped
- 1 apple, cored and slice
- ¼ tsp salt
- chopped nuts, dried cranberries, garnish (optional)

DIRECTIONS

1. Add all the ingredients to a bowl before mixing and seasoning to taste.
2. Set out the apple slices before spooning the mixture on top and enjoy.

Chicken Fricassee

A delicious chicken stew with earthy undertones that will soon become a new winter favorite. As the dish bubbles away in your kitchen, enjoy the scents of leeks, as you prepare to dish a large bowl of comfort. While not traditionally Mediterranean by origin (it's a French dish), the ingredients and overall flavor profile align with Mediterranean favorites.

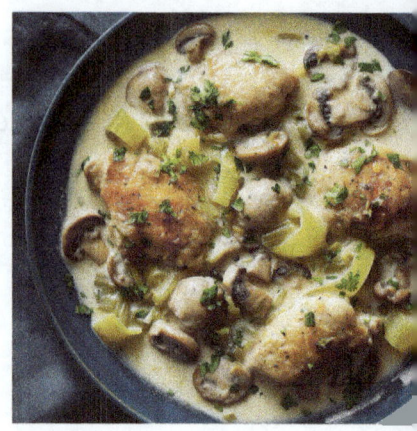

TIME: 50 MIN	SERVINGS: 4	PREP: 10 MIN	COOK: 40 MIN
CALORIES: 306 KCAL	CARBS: 16.5 G	FAT: 16 G	PROTEIN: 26.8 G

INGREDIENTS

- 1 tbsp olive oil
- 2 tbsp paleo sour cream (made with coconut milk and lemon juice)
- 6 cups white button mushrooms, rinsed and quartered
- 1 tbsp almond flour
- 1 cup leeks, rinsed and diced
- 1 tbsp lemon juice
- 2 tbsp fresh parsley
- 1 cup celery, rinsed and diced
- 3 cup chicken broth, homemade with no thickening agent
- 1 cup onion, peeled and diced
- 1 lb chicken thighs, skinless
- ¼ tsp ground black pepper
- ½ tsp salt

DIRECTIONS

1. Preheat the oven to 350 °F.
2. Add some olive oil to a sauté pan, and heat to medium.
3. Cook the mushrooms for 3–5 minutes before adding the onions, leeks, and celery, and cook for another 3–5 minutes.
4. Pour in the chicken broth and boil before adding the thighs. Cover with an oven-safe lid and move the pan into the oven to bake for 20 minutes or until the chicken is cooked.
5. Place the pan on the stovetop, remove the meat, and add the herbs and lemon juice before boiling.
6. In a bowl, whisk the paleo sour cream and almond flour before pouring it into the pan on the stovetop. Allow the mixture to boil once more before removing it from the heat.
7. Pour the mixture from the pan between 4 bowls and top with a ¼ of prepared chicken.

Mediterranean-Paleo Chicken Skillet

With a combination of tomatoes, artichokes, and olives, you'll be hard-pressed to find a more Mediterranean dish that is as filling and tasty without any pasta added. To save time with the recipe, you can buy precooked chicken.

TIME: 25 MIN	SERVINGS: 4	PREP: 10 MIN	COOK: 15 MIN
CALORIES: 358 KCAL	CARBS: 22.1 G	FAT: 11.6 G	PROTEIN: 4.6 G

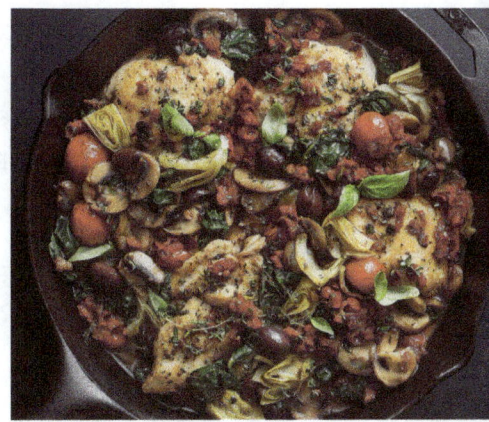

INGREDIENTS

- ½ cup sun-dried tomatoes, chopped
- ¼ tsp pepper
- ½ yellow onion, diced
- ¼ tsp salt
- 2-3 cloves garlic, minced
- 1 tsp dried oregano
- 8 oz mushrooms, sliced
- 1 tsp dried parsley
- 3 Roma tomatoes, diced
- 1 tbsp balsamic vinegar
- 8 oz jarred artichoke hearts, liquid drained
- 2-3 tbsp olive oil
- ⅓ cup kalamata olives, chopped
- 2 handfuls fresh spinach leaves
- 1 lb pre-cooked chicken breasts, chopped
- 2 tbsp fresh basil, for garnish (optional)

DIRECTIONS

1. Add the onion and a tablespoon of oil to a skillet and bring the heat up to medium. Sauté the onion for 3–4 minutes.
2. Add the garlic and cook for another minute before adding the sliced mushrooms to cook for 5–7 minutes. Season to taste.
3. Pour a tablespoon of olive oil and balsamic vinegar before adding the olives, artichoke hearts, fresh and dried tomatoes, oregano, and parsley, and then stir for a few minutes.
4. Place the spinach and the chicken in the pan, stir, and cook for another 1–2 minutes.
5. Season as needed and serve hot with some fresh basil.

Braised Cod with Leeks

Cod makes a lightly flavored Mediterranean fish dish that is truly enhanced when cooked in chicken stock. With mild-flavored leeks, the fish will surely take center stage when served. Enjoy as is or served on a bed of steamed collard greens (see Mediterranean Marinated Tenderloin recipe).

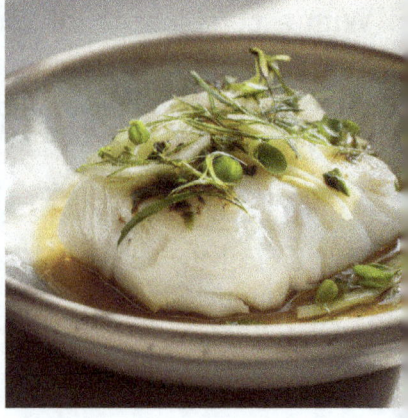

TIME: 40 MIN	SERVINGS: 4	PREP: 10 MIN	COOK: 30 MIN
CALORIES: 309 KCAL	CARBS: 45.3 G	FAT: 4.8 G	PROTEIN: 22.8 G

INGREDIENTS

- 2 cup leeks, split lengthwise and sliced thin
- 2 cups chicken broth, homemade
- 3 carrots, peeled, and cut into thin sticks
- 12 oz cod filet, divided into 4 portions
- 2 tbsp fresh parsley, chopped
- ¼ tsp ground black pepper
- ½ tsp salt
- 1 tbsp coconut oil

DIRECTIONS

1. In a sauté pan, add the coconut oil and the fish. Cook for 3 minutes a side and remove.
2. Stir in the carrots and leeks, then cook for 3–5 minutes until soft.
3. Pour in the broth, salt, parsley, pepper, and raise the temperature to high to bring to a boil. Lower the heat until a simmer is reached.
4. Simmer the mixture for 10–12 minutes until vegetables are tender.
5. Replace the fish and cover the pan. Keep the temperature low and cook the mixture for 5 minutes until the fish flakes easily.
6. Serve warm.

Meatballs and Zoodles

This meal is so tasty, you won't ever miss noodles again. The zoodles, meatballs, and the tomato mixture are each created separately before being joined, making it a meal that can easily be prepared ahead of time. Plus, the entire meal can be frozen for later use. It only takes 6 minutes to reheat.

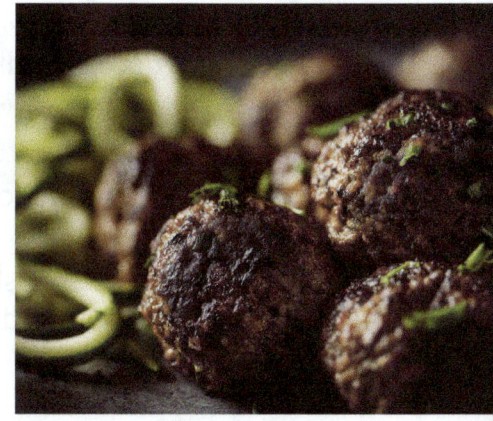

TIME: 50 MIN	SERVINGS: 4	PREP: 20 MIN	COOK: 30 MIN
CALORIES: 401 KCAL	CARBS: 21.7 G	FAT: 26.9 G	PROTEIN: 27.5 G

INGREDIENTS

FOR THE MEATBALLS:
- 1 large egg
- 1 lb ground beef
- 1 tsp coconut aminos
- 2 cloves of garlic, crushed
- 1 tsp balsamic vinegar
- 1 small onion, minced
- ½ tsp parsley dried
- 1 tbsp coconut flour
- ¼ tsp pepper
- ½ tsp salt
- ½ tsp basil
- 2 tbsp coconut oil
- ½ tsp oregano

FOR THE TOMATOES:
- 2 tbsp olive oil
- ½ teaspoon basil
- 2 pints of grape tomatoes
- ½ teaspoon salt
- 2 cloves of garlic, crushed
- ½ teaspoon oregano

FOR THE ZOODLES:
- 3 medium zucchini, spiralized (directions in Chicken and Zoodles with Pesto recipe)

DIRECTIONS

Meatballs:
1. Preheat the oven to 350°F.
2. Combine all meatball ingredients (except the coconut oil) in a mixing bowl. Let the mixture rest for 5 minutes.
3. Heat the coconut oil in an oven-safe skillet over medium heat.
4. Form the meat mixture into small balls and place them in the skillet. Brown the meatballs on all sides.
5. Transfer the skillet to the oven and bake for 10 minutes, or until the meatballs are cooked through.

Tomatoes:
1. Heat olive oil in a large skillet over medium heat.
2. Add the grape tomatoes, crushed garlic, basil, oregano, and salt.
3. Cook, stirring occasionally, until the tomatoes soften and begin to burst, about 8-10 minutes.

Zoodles:
1. Spiralize 3 medium zucchini using a spiralizer (refer to the Chicken and Zoodles with Pesto recipe for details).
2. Add the zoodles to the skillet with the cooked tomatoes and toss gently to combine. Cook for 2-3 minutes until heated through but still slightly firm.

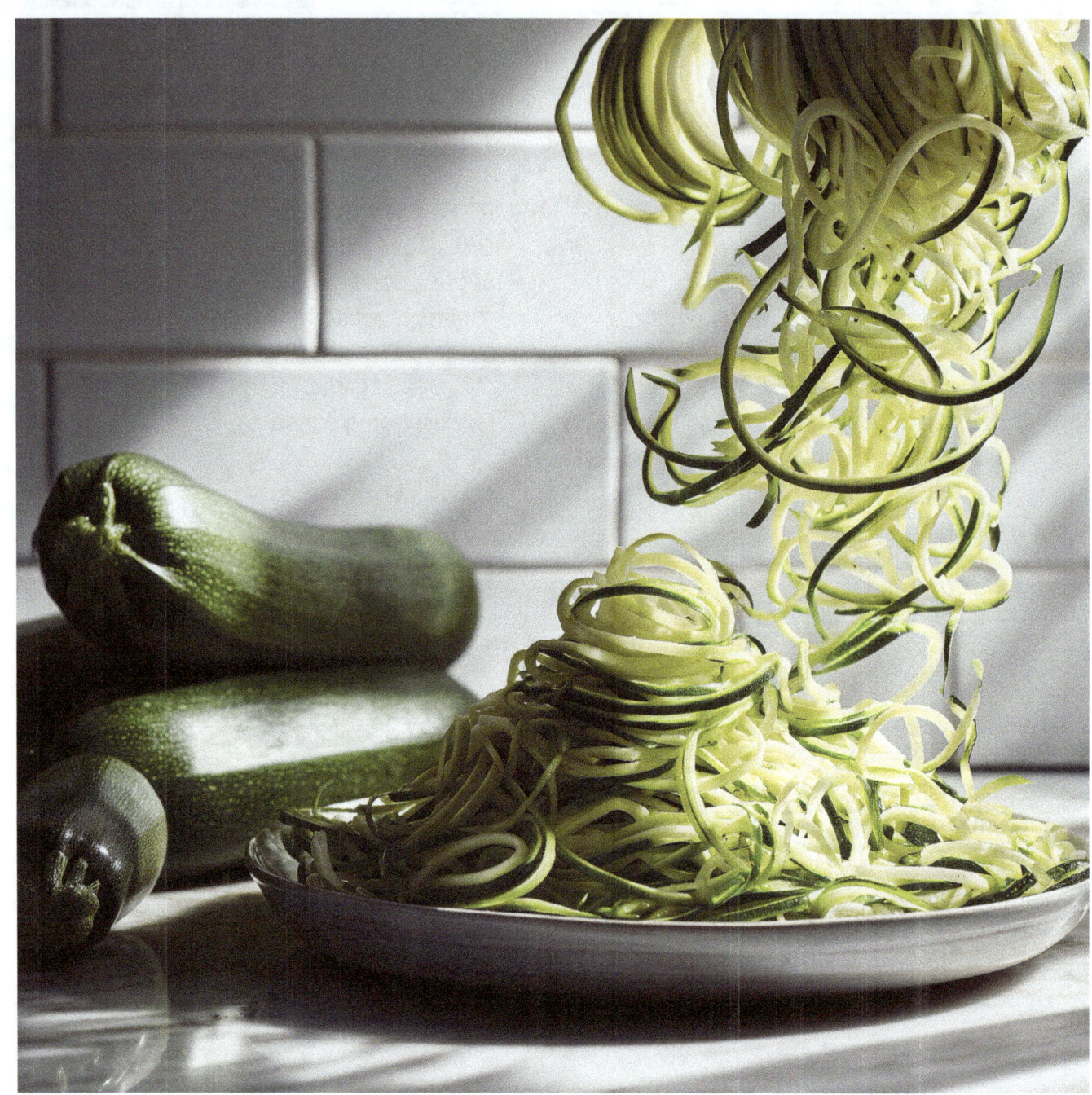

Pork Filet with Apple Sauce

While apples, walnuts, raisins, and cinnamon are often associated with dessert, they add a unique blend of sweet and strong flavors to create a homemade sauce perfect for pork (or substitute with beef tenderloin). Once ready, pour the apple sauce over some perfectly broiled pork tenderloin to create a taste sensation. Serve on a bed of arugula.

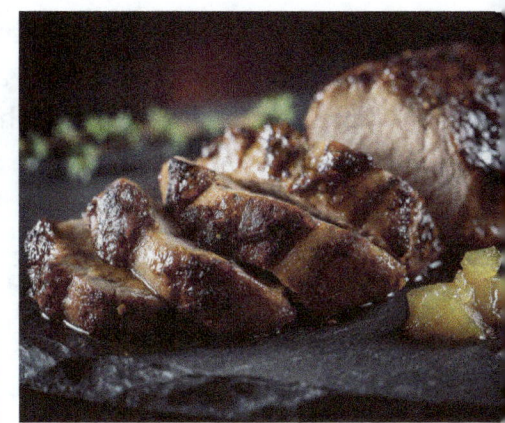

TIME: 30 MIN	SERVINGS: 4	PREP: 10 MIN	COOK: 20 MIN
CALORIES: 365 KCAL	CARBS: 4.8 G	FAT: 10.3 G	PROTEIN: 60.5 G

INGREDIENTS

- ½ tsp ground cinnamon
- 2 tbsp raisins
- 2 apples, cored, not peeled, cut into ¼-inch pieces from bottom up
- ⅛ tsp ground black pepper
- 2 lb pork tenderloin (or substitute with beef tenderloin)
- 2 tbsp walnuts, crushed
- ¼ tsp salt

DIRECTIONS

1. Set the oven rack within 3 inches from the element and preheat the broiler on high.
2. Place aluminum foil inside a broiler pan and lightly coat it with olive oil.
3. Cut 8 pork rounds from the center of the pork tenderloins to be 1 ½-inch thick, saving the ends for a different meal.
4. Add the pork rounds to the broiler pan and season, then set aside until the oven is at temperature.
5. Broil the meat for 5–10 minutes on each side, ensuring they're cooked through.
6. As the meat cooks, add ½ cup of water to a pan and bring it to a boil.
7. Add the apple slices, walnuts, raisins, and cinnamon to the pan before lowering the heat to medium.
8. Cover the pan and allow the mixture to simmer, until the fruit starts to soften and the apple can easily be pierced.
9. Once soft enough, remove from the heat and pour over each serving of precut tenderloins.

Easy and Delicious Shrimp Sheet Pan

Enjoy the classic tastes of the Mediterranean with this shrimp sheet meal bursting with flavors and textures from tomatoes, artichokes, olives, and onions. The crushed red pepper is a must to bring a hint of spiciness to the dish.

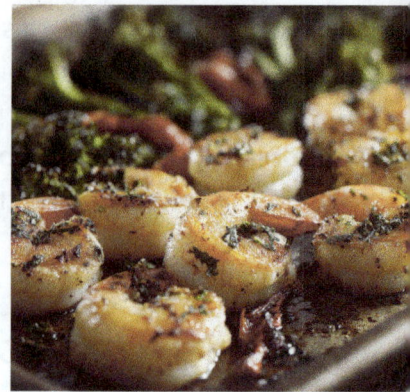

TIME: 45 MIN	SERVINGS: 4	PREP: 25 MIN	COOK: 20 MIN
CALORIES: 328 KCAL	CARBS: 17 G	FAT: 16 G	PROTEIN: 29 G

INGREDIENTS

FOR VEGETABLES:
- 1 tsp dried oregano
- 1 medium lemon zest
- 1 tsp kosher salt
- 1 red onion, cut into ½-inch slices
- 12–14 oz canned artichoke hearts, quartered and drained
- 3–4 tbsp lemon juice, divided
- 3 cloves garlic, minced
- ¼ cup kalamata olives, pitted and coarsely chopped
- 1 pint grape tomatoes
- 1 ½ tbsp olive oil
- ¼ tsp black pepper
- 1 medium zucchini, trimmed, sliced lengthwise, and cut in ½-inch pieces

FOR SHRIMPS:
- 1 tbsp lemon juice
- 1 tbsp olive oil
- ¼ tsp dried oregano
- ¼ tsp crushed red pepper
- ¼ tsp kosher salt
- 1 lb jumbo raw shrimp, peeled and deveined
- 2 tbsp fresh parsley, chopped

DIRECTIONS

1. Preheat the oven to 450 °F.
2. Place some parchment paper in a large-rimmed baking tray.
3. In a large bowl, add a tablespoon of lemon juice, all the spices, and garlic before whisking well.
4. Add in all the vegetables and toss until well-coated.
5. Pour the mixture into the baking tray, keeping the vegetables in a single layer, then adding it to the oven to bake for 12 minutes. Move on to preparing the shrimp.
6. In the same bowl, add the remaining lemon juice, shrimp spices, and the shrimp before tossing well.
7. Once the vegetables are cooked, remove them from the oven, and add the shrimp (avoiding adding any excess liquid). Stir the shrimp and vegetables together before spreading the mixture out in a single layer.
8. Place the tray back in the oven and cook for another 6–10 minutes until the shrimp become pink. Don't overcook.
9. Once cooked, sprinkle a tablespoon of lemon juice and parsley over the mixture and serve with a side of potatoes and fresh Greek salad. Season to your preference.

REFERENCES

Ambitious Kitchen. (2021, April 5). Healthy lemon bars (gluten free, dairy free & paleo!). https://www.ambitiouskitchen.com/healthy-lemon-bars-gluten-free-dairy-free-paleo/

Anderson, J. (2020, January 29). Getting started with the gluten-free diet. Verywell Fit. https://www.verywellfit.com/gluten-free-diet-grocery-lists-recipes-and-more-4691786

Baker, S. (2020, September 4). Easy keto meal planning tips: Keto meal prep ideas. Nutiro. https://my.nutiro.com/keto-meal-prep-ideas/

Baker, S. (2021a, January 4). The best tips to start a vegetarian meal plan. Nutiro. https://my.nutiro.com/vegetarian-meal-plan/

Baker, S. (2021b, February 8). Paleo diet to lose weight. Nutiro. https://my.nutiro.com/paleo-diet-to-lose-weight/

Bandurski, K. (2021, February 2). The ultimate 7-day vegetarian meal plan for anyone trying to eat less meat. Taste of Home. https://www.tasteofhome.com/collection/vegetarian-meal-plan/

Bashinsky, R. (2022, May). Chickpea & roasted red pepper lettuce wraps with tahini dressing. EatingWell. https://www.eatingwell.com/recipe/269835/chickpea-roasted-red-pepper-lettuce-wraps-with-tahini-dressing/

Beauty Bites. (2022, June 29). 30+ meal prep Mediterranean diet recipes. https://www.beautybites.org/meal-prep-mediterranean-diet-recipes/

Best, C. (2014a, October). Speedy Mediterranean gnocchi. BBC Good Food. https://www.bbcgoodfood.com/recipes/speedy-mediterranean-gnocchi

Best, C. (2014b, November). Spanish meatball & butter bean stew. BBC Good Food. https://www.bbcgoodfood.com/recipes/spanish-meatball-butter-bean-stew

Bradley, B. (2018a, March 23). Italian polenta pizza with caramelized onions. Mediterranean Living. https://www.mediterraneanliving.com/italian-polenta-pizza-with-caramelized-onions-and-kalamata-olives-gluten-free/

Bradley, B. (2018b, July 7). Grilled salmon salad with yogurt dill dressing. Mediterranean Living. https://www.mediterraneanliving.com/grilled-salmon-salad-with-yogurt-dill-dressing/

Bryan, L. (2016, March 25). Rosemary grilled lamb chops with mint apple sauce. Downshiftology. https://downshiftology.com/recipes/rosemary-grilled-lamb-chops-mint-apple-sauce/

Bryan, L. (2017, October 19). Tahini recipe (super easy & creamy). Downshiftology. https://downshiftology.com/recipes/tahini/

Bryan, L. (2018a, August 18). Smoked salmon, avocado and cucumber bites. Downshiftology. https://downshiftology.com/recipes/smoked-salmon-avocado-cucumber-bites/

Bryan, L. (2018b, December 19). Shakshuka. Downshiftology. https://downshiftology.com/recipes/shakshuka/

Cadogan, M. (2014, August). All-in-one fish supper. BBC Good Food. https://www.bbcgoodfood.com/recipes/all-one-fish-supper

Casner, C. (2018, June). Tomato, cucumber & white-bean salad with basil vinaigrette. EatingWell. https://www.eatingwell.com/recipe/265886/tomato-cucumber-white-bean-salad-with-basil-vinaigrette/

Casner, C. (2019, February). Gluten-Free morning glory blender muffins. EatingWell. https://www.eatingwell.com/recipe/270874/gluten-free-morning-glory-blender-muffins/

Casner, C. (n.d.). Chicken quinoa bowl with olives & cucumber. EatingWell. https://www.eatingwell.com/recipe/255217/chicken-quinoa-bowl-with-olives-cucumbers/

Cast Iron Keto. (2018, February 8). Mediterranean keto shrimp zoodles. https://www.castironketo.net/blog/mediterranean-keto-shrimp-zoodles

Christala. (2022, July 29). Branzino Mediterranean. Allrecipes. https://www.allrecipes.com/recipe/236932/branzino-mediterranean/

Clarke, E. (2021, April 5). Sheet pan Mediterranean shrimp. Well Plated by Erin. https://www.wellplated.com/sheet-pan-mediterranean-shrimp

Cleveland Clinic. (2022, November 20). Mediterranean diet. https://my.clevelandclinic.org/health/articles/16037-mediterranean-diet

Cook For Your Life. (n.d.). Steamed collard greens. https://www.cookforyourlife.org/recipes/steamed-collard-greens/

Dansky, L. (2021, March). Quinoa salad with feta, olives & tomatoes. EatingWell. https://www.eatingwell.com/recipe/7893499/quinoa-salad-feta-olives-tomatoes/

Denise. (2016, January 16). Paleo meatballs with zoodles (freezable healthy lunches). My Life Cookbook. https://mylifecookbook.com/paleo-meatballs-with-zoodles-freezable-healthy-lunches/

EatingWell Test Kitchen. (2018, December). Fig & ricotta overnight oats. EatingWell. https://www.eatingwell.com/recipe/269659/fig-ricotta-overnight-oats/

EatingWell Test Kitchen. (n.d.). Mediterranean veggie wrap with cilantro hummus. EatingWell. https://www.eatingwell.com/recipe/266299/mediterranean-veggie-wrap-with-cilantro-hummus/

Florian. (2020, August 17). 10 minute Mediterranean vegan pasta. Contentedness Cooking. https://www.contentednesscooking.com/10-minute-mediterranean-vegan-pasta/

Fusion Craftiness. (2016, September 13). Creamy French scrambled eggs recipe | oeufs brouilles. https://www.fusioncraftiness.com/creamy-french-scrambled-eggs-recipe-oeufs-brouilles/

Good Food team. (2002, August). Silvana's Mediterranean & basil pasta. BBC Good Food. https://www.bbcgoodfood.com/recipes/silvanas-mediterranean-basil-pasta

Good Food team. (2012, June). Pancetta-wrapped fish with lemony potatoes. BBC Good Food. https://www.bbcgoodfood.com/recipes/pancetta-wrapped-fish-lemony-potatoes

Gunaydin, Z., & Gunaydin, Y. (2019, October 16). Mediterranean green olive salad. Give Recipe. https://www.giverecipe.com/green-olive-salad-for-breakfast

Gunnars, K. (2021, October 25). Mediterranean diet 101: A meal plan and beginner's guide. Healthline. https://www.healthline.com/nutrition/mediterranean-diet-meal-plan#the-basics

Gunnars, K. (2022, November 29). The paleo diet — A beginner's guide plus meal plan. Healthline. https://www.healthline.com/nutrition/paleo-diet-meal-plan-and-menu

Haas, S. (2016). Salmon pita sandwich. EatingWell. https://www.eatingwell.com/recipe/255162/salmon-pita-sandwich

Hart, E. (2021, February 22). Red tomato pesto. Erren's Kitchen. https://www.errenskitchen.com/red-tomato-pesto/

Hendley, J. (2019, May). Mascarpone & berries toast. EatingWell. https://www.eatingwell.com/recipe/272746/mascarpone-berries-toast/

Her Highness, Hungry Me. (2020, August 20). Mediterranean eggs breakfast bowl recipe. https://hh-hm.com/mediterranean-eggs-breakfast-bowl-recipe/

Jawad, Y. (2022, August 18). Mediterranean hummus bowl. FeelGoodFoodie. https://feelgoodfoodie.net/recipe/mediterranean-hummus-bowl/

Johnson, A. (2022, November 8). 15 Mediterranean herbs, spices & seasonings every cook needs. Medmunch. https://medmunch.com/mediterranean-spices/

Kanya, L. (2022, October). Lemon ricotta pancakes. EatingWell. https://www.eatingwell.com/recipe/8009783/lemon-ricotta-pancakes/

Kapsalis, R. (2021, December 20). Mediterranean low carb example – seafood stew with a handful of veggies. Greek Goes Keto. https://www.greekgoesketo.com/mediterranean-stew

Karadsheh, S. (2020, April 26). Grilled swordfish recipe with a Mediterranean twist. The Mediterranean Dish. https://www.themediterraneandish.com/grilled-swordfish-recipe/

Karadsheh, S. (2021, January 4). Complete Mediterranean diet shopping list. The Mediterranean Dish. https://www.themediterraneandish.com/mediterranean-diet-shopping-list/

Karadsheh, S. (2021b, December 1). Burbara (wheat berry pudding). The Mediterranean Dish. https://www.themediterraneandish.com/burbara-wheat-berry-pudding/

Kelly. (2021, February 4). Baked feta pasta. Life Made Sweeter. https://lifemadesweeter.com/baked-feta-pasta

Killeen, B. (2022, June). Cucumber, tomato & arugula salad with hummus. EatingWell. https://www.eatingwell.com/recipe/258521/cucumber-tomato-arugula-salad-with-hummus/

Lachtrupp, E. (2022, November 22). Vegan meal plan for beginners. EatingWell. https://www.eatingwell.com/article/7902516/vegan-meal-plan-for-beginners/

Laughlin, J. (2022, April 21). Greek quinoa bowls. Peas and Crayons. https://peasandcrayons.com/2016/01/greek-quinoa-bowls-recipe.html

Leanne. (2019, August 15). Mediterranean quiche with almond crust. Crumb Top Baking. https://www.crumbtopbaking.com/mediterranean-quiche/

Lester, L. (2020, March 26). Keto Mediterranean chicken skillet. KetoDiet. https://ketodietapp.com/Blog/lchf/keto-mediterranean-chicken-skillet

Lexi. (2020, September 28). Mediterranean grilled tofu. Crowded Kitchen. https://www.crowdedkitchen.com/mediterranean-grilled-tofu

Lolley, P. (2021, April). Lentil salad with feta, tomatoes, cucumbers & olives. EatingWell. https://www.eatingwell.com/recipe/7899362/lentil-salad-with-feta-tomatoes-cucumbers-olives/

Love2Teach. (n.d.). Rib-Eye steaks with Mediterranean marinade recipe. Food. https://www.food.com/recipe/rib-eye-steaks-with-mediterranean-marinade-169971

Macey, D. (2022, May 26). Vegan grocery list. Running on Real Food. https://runningonrealfood.com/vegan-grocery-list/

Malcoun, C. (2018, December). Berry chia pudding. EatingWell. https://www.eatingwell.com/recipe/268739/berry-chia-pudding/

Mawer, R. (2020, October 22). The ketogenic diet: A detailed beginner's guide to keto. Healthline. https://www.healthline.com/nutrition/ketogenic-diet-101

Mayo Clinic Staff. (2021, December 11). Gluten-free diet. Mayo Clinic. https://www.mayoclinic.org/healthy-lifestyle/nutrition-and-healthy-eating/in-depth/gluten-free-diet/art-20048530

Meyer, H. (2018, March). Meal-prep roasted vegetable bowls with pesto. EatingWell. https://www.eatingwell.com/recipe/263548/meal-prep-roasted-vegetable-bowls-with-pesto/

Migala, J. (2022, August 2). What is the Mediterranean diet? A detailed beginner's guide. Everyday Health. https://www.everydayhealth.com/mediterranean-diet/guide/

Moore, A. (2020, May 6). These are the standard macronutrients on a Mediterranean diet plate. MindBodyGreen. https://www.mindbodygreen.com/articles/mediterranean-diet-macros

Moreno, J. (2018, September 27). Harissa chickpea stew with eggplant and millet. PureWow. https://www.purewow.com/recipes/harissa-chickpea-stew-eggplant-millet

Neil. (2022, September 3). Mediterranean breakfast egg muffins. Neils Healthy Meals. https://neilshealthymeals.com/mediterranean-breakfast-egg-muffins/

Nutiro. (2021, February 4). Shopping list when starting keto diet and what you need to know. https://nutiro.com/keto-shopping-list/

Nutiro. (2022a, May 3). The best breakfast muffins – keto meal prep ideas. https://nutiro.com/keto-breakfast-muffins/

Nutiro. (2022b, May 25). Quinoa rice pilaf with dried cherries and toasted pine nuts. https://nutiro.com/quinoa-rice-pilaf-with-dried-cherries-and-toasted-pine-nuts/

Nutiro. (2022c, May 26). Chicken penne pasta and broccoli with cheese melts. https://nutiro.com/chic-penne-pasta-and-broccoli-with-cheese-melts/

Nutiro. (2022d, May 26). Spanish frittata with cubed potatoes. https://nutiro.com/spanish-frittata-with-cubed-potatoes/

Nutiro. (2022e, May 27). One of the saffron lamb tagines you'll love. https://nutiro.com/one-of-the-saffron-lamb-tagines-youll-love/

Nutiro. (2022f, May 27). Sesame chicken recipe with peppers and snow peas. https://nutiro.com/sesame-chicken-recipe-with-peppers-and-snow-peas/

Nutiro. (2022g, May 27). Smoked salmon and feta fritters make with dipping sauce. https://nutiro.com/smoked-salmon-and-feta-fritters-make-with-dipping-sauce/

Nutiro. (2022h, May 28). Orecchiette with creamy basil and broccoli sauce. https://nutiro.com/orecchiette-with-creamy-basil-and-broccoli-sauce/

Nutiro. (2022i, May 28). Roasted chicken, vegetable and Risoni salad you'll love. https://nutiro.com/roasted-chicken-vegetable-and-risoni-salad-youll-love/

Nutiro. (2022j, May 28). Zesty oriental chicken salad you'll love. https://nutiro.com/zesty-oriental-chicken-salad/

Nutiro. (2022k, May 29). Dijon glazed and herb crusted potato salad you'll love. https://nutiro.com/dijon-glazed-and-herb-crusted-potato-salad/

Nutiro. (2022l, May 30). Satisfy me and look no more almond butter keto cupcake. https://nutiro.com/satisfy-me-and-look-no-more-almond-butter-keto-cupcake/

Nutiro. (2022m, May 31). Broccoli and firm tofu recipe you'll love. https://nutiro.com/broccoli-and-firm-tofu-recipe/

Nutiro. (2022n, May 31). Cheesy tomato omelet with mozzarella. https://nutiro.com/cheesy-tomato-omelet-with-mozzarella/

Nutiro. (2022o, May 31). Chicken fricassee recipe with mushrooms. https://nutiro.com/chicken-fricassee-recipe-with-mushrooms/

Nutiro. (2022p, May 31). Easy ground turkey skillet recipe made in one pan. https://nutiro.com/easy-ground-turkey-skillet-recipe-made-in-one-pan/

Nutiro. (2022q, May 31). Easy no bake cookies recipe with coconut. https://nutiro.com/easy-no-bake-cookies-recipe-with-coconut/

Nutiro. (2022r, June 2). Gluten free non insalata caprese pasta recipe. https://nutiro.com/gluten-free-non-insalata-caprese-pasta-recipe/

Nutiro. (2022s, June 2). Grilled pork tenderloin with a southeast asian marinade. https://nutiro.com/grilled-pork-tenderloin-with-a-southeast-asian-marinade/

Nutiro. (2022t, June 2). Pork filet mignon with french applesauce recipe you'll love. https://nutiro.com/pork-filet-mignon-with-french-applesauce-recipe-youll-love/

Nutiro. (2022u, June 4). Braised cod with leeks and crisp potatoes. https://nutiro.com/braised-cod-with-leeks-and-crisp-potatoes/

Nutiro. (2022v, June 4). Recipe for quinoa and kale stew with red lentils. https://nutiro.com/recipe-for-quinoa-and-kale-stew-with-red-lentils/

Nutiro. (2022w, June 6). Chicken salad recipe with tangy tomatillo and cilantro. https://nutiro.com/chicken-salad-recipe-with-tangy-tomatillo-and-cilantro/

Nutiro. (2022x, June 6). Chocolate keto cupcakes recipe you'll love. https://nutiro.com/chocolate-keto-cupcakes-recipe/

Nutiro. (2022y, June 6). Easy Moroccan chicken stew with or without couscous. https://nutiro.com/moroccan-chicken-stew-with-couscous/

Nutiro. (2022z, June 6). Grilled tuna with baby spinach salad with chickpeas. https://nutiro.com/grilled-tuna-baby-spinach-salad-with-chickpeas/

Nutiro. (2022aa, June 6). Mediterranean beef and marinated chicken kabobs on the grill. https://nutiro.com/mediterranean-marinated-chicken-kabobs-on-the-grill/

Nutiro. (2022ab, June 8). Avocado pesto pasta with chicken and zucchini spaghetti recipe. https://nutiro.com/avocado-pesto-pasta-with-chicken-and-zucchini-spaghetti-recipe/

Nutiro. (2022ac, June 8). Stuffed avocados with chicken recipe you'll love. https://nutiro.com/stuffed-avocados-with-chicken-recipe-youll-love/

Nutiro. (2022ad, June 11). Easy chicken salad recipe with avocado oil healthy mayo. https://nutiro.com/easy-chicken-salad-recipe-with-avocado-oil-healthy-mayo/

Nutiro. (2022ae, June 11). Easy Spanish style feta cheese keto frittata recipe. https://nutiro.com/easy-spanish-style-feta-cheese-keto-frittata-recipe/

O'Brien, D. (2016, December). Roasted beet hummus. EatingWell. https://www.eatingwell.com/recipe/256574/roasted-beet-hummus/

Oldways. (2016, April 14). What does breakfast in the Mediterranean look like? https://oldwayspt.org/blog/what-does-breakfast-mediterranean-look

Oldways. (2018, May 8). The nutty and seedy side of the Mediterranean diet. https://oldwayspt.org/blog/nutty-and-seedy-side-mediterranean-diet

Oldways. (2019a). Traditional Med diet. https://oldwayspt.org/traditional-diets/mediterranean-diet/traditional-med-diet

Oldways. (2019b, March 25). Your guide to Mediterranean spices. https://oldwayspt.org/blog/your-guide-mediterranean-spices

Oldways. (2022, January 5). Whole grains with a mediterranean flair. https://wholegrainscouncil.org/blog/2022/01/whole-grains-mediterranean-flair

Oldways. (n.d.-a). Chickpea hash & eggs. https://oldwayspt.org/recipes/chickpea-hash-eggs

Oldways. (n.d.-b). Oldways homemade granola. https://oldwayspt.org/recipes/oldways-homemade-granola

Petre, A. (2022, May 12). The vegan diet: A complete guide for beginners. Healthline. https://www.healthline.com/nutrition/vegan-diet-guide

PureWow Editors. (2015, August 20). Stuffed eggplant. PureWow. https://www.purewow.com/recipes/Stuffed-Eggplant

PureWow Editors. (2018a, August 3). Wild alaska salmon and smashed cucumber grain bowls. PureWow. https://www.purewow.com/recipes/wild-alaska-salmon-cucumber-grain-bowls

PureWow Editors. (2018b, September 26). Pesto quinoa bowls with roasted veggies and labneh. PureWow. https://www.purewow.com/recipes/pesto-quinoa-bowl-roasted-veggies-labneh

Raman, R., & Link, R. (2022, July 31). The gluten-free diet: A beginner's guide with meal plan. Healthline. https://www.healthline.com/nutrition/gluten-free-diet

Reynolds, H. B. (n.d.). Muffin pan frittatas. Oldways. https://oldwayspt.org/recipes/muffin-pan-frittatas

Rivers, A. (2021, January 21). Creamy tuscan garlic chicken. The Recipe Critic. https://therecipecritic.com/creamy-tuscan-garlic-chicken

Seaver, V. (2017, November). Yogurt with blueberries & honey. EatingWell. https://www.eatingwell.com/recipe/261617/yogurt-with-blueberries-honey/

Seaver, V. (2018, May). Prosciutto, mozzarella & melon plate. EatingWell. https://www.eatingwell.com/recipe/264491/prosciutto-mozzarella-melon-plate/

Sissom, B. (2019, May 6). Make ahead fruit and yogurt parfaits (video). Simply Sissom. https://www.simplysissom.com/simpleyogurtparfaits/

Stephanie. (2016, April 14). Apple tuna bites. Eat. Drink. Love. https://eat-drink-love.com/apple-tuna-bites/

Trina. (n.d.). One skillet paleo mediterranean chicken recipe. Paleo Newbie. https://www.paleonewbie.com/one-skillet-paleo-mediterranean-chicken/

Unify Health Team. (2020, March 2). Try this vegetarian grocery list for beginners: Essential vegetarian shopping list. Unify. https://unifyhealthlabs.com/vegetarian-grocery-list-beginners/

Webber, J. (2017, December 26). A paleo shopping list for beginners (so you're not tempted to buy bread). Greatist. https://greatist.com/eat/paleo-shopping-list#1

Webster, K. (2017, August). Quinoa chickpea salad with roasted red pepper hummus dressing. EatingWell. https://www.eatingwell.com/recipe/259996/quinoa-chickpea-salad-with-roasted-red-pepper-hummus-dressing/

Winn, J., & Winn, E. (2020, October 5). Mediterranean breakfast frittata (paleo, whole30 + keto). Real Simple Good. https://realsimplegood.com/mediterranean-breakfast-frittata/

The Whole Cook. (2022, November 14). Easy homemade Italian dressing. The Whole Cook. https://thewholecook.com/easy-homemade-italian-dressing/

Zisk, J. (2022, February 15). Greek salad recipe. One Dish Kitchen. https://onedishkitchen.com/greek-salad-recipe/

INDEX

CHICKEN
- Chicken Fricassee - Page 118
- Chicken Penne with Broccoli and Cheese - Page 35
- Chicken Quinoa Bowl - Page 40
- Chicken Salad with Cilantro and Tomatoes - Page 37
- Chicken and Pesto Zoodles - Page 69
- Chicken, Vegetables, and Risoni Salad - Page 20
- Marinated Chicken and Beef Kabobs - Page 14
- Mediterranean Chicken Salad - Page 68
- Mediterranean-Paleo Chicken Skillet - Page 119
- Moroccan Chicken Stew - Page 80
- One Skillet Greek Isle Chicken - Page 71
- Sesame Chicken with Snap Peas and Peppers - Page 18
- Turkey Skillet Meal - Page 85
- Tuscan Garlic Chicken - Page 73
- Zesty Mediterranean Chicken Salad - Page 114

BEEF
- Meatballs and Zoodles - Page 121
- Mediterranean Marinated Tenderloin - Page 27
- Spanish Meatball and Bean Stew - Page 25

SEAFOOD
- All-In-One Fish Supper - Page 22
- Apple Tuna Bites - Page 117
- Easy and Delicious Shrimp Sheet Pan - Page 124
- Fish and Lemony Potatoes - Page 26
- Grilled Salmon Salad - Page 81
- Grilled Tuna with Spinach and Chickpeas - Page 29
- Salmon Pita - Page 41
- Salmon and Cucumber Bowl - Page 36
- Salmon, Cucumber, and Avocado Bites - Page 55
- Seafood Stew - Page 72
- Shrimp Zoodles - Page 79
- Smoked Salmon and Feta Fritters - Page 13
- Spanish Paella - Page 17

LAMB
- Rosemary Grilled Lamb Chops - Page 24
- Saffron Lamb Tagine - Page 23

PORK
- Pork Filet with Apple Sauce - Page 123

VEGETARIAN (DAIRY/EGGS)
- Baked Feta Pasta - Page 111
- Chickpea Hash and Eggs - Page 48
- Greek Moussaka - Page 15
- Greek Yogurt Parfait - Page 105
- Mediterranean Egg Bowl - Page 77
- Mediterranean Egg Muffins - Page 50
- Stuffed Eggplant - Page 33

PLANT-BASED (VEGAN)
- Beet Hummus - Page 60
- Broccoli and Tofu - Page 90
- Greek Salad with Hummus - Page 108
- Mediterranean Grill Tofu - Page 104
- Mediterranean Hummus Bowl - Page 92
- Mediterranean Vegan Pasta - Page 99
- Roasted Red Pepper Hummus with Quinoa Chickpea Salad - Page 98
- Vegan-Friendly Pilaf - Page 91
- Veggie Wrap with Cilantro Hummus - Page 109

PASTA
- Caprese Pasta Salad - Page 84
- Mediterranean Gnocchi - Page 19
- Mediterranean and Basil Pasta - Page 21
- Orecchiette With Broccoli and Basil Sauce - Page 106

BREAKFAST
- Berry Chia Pudding - Page 51
- Fig and Ricotta Overnight Oats - Page 49
- Keto Breakfast Muffins - Page 64
- Lemon Ricotta Pancakes - Page 103
- Mozzarella Omelet - Page 102
- Muffin Frittatas - Page 46
- Oeufs Brouillés - Page 45
- Paleo-Mediterranean Frittata - Page 115
- Shakshuka - Page 52

SNACK
- Almond Butter Mug Cake - Page 57
- Chocolate Cupcakes - Page 56
- Mascarpone and Berries Toast - Page 58
- No Bake Coconut Cookies - Page 54
- Sweet and Savory Mezze Platter - Page 61
- Yogurt With Blueberries and Honey - Page 59
- Zesty Lemon Bars - Page 116

BREAKFAST/SNACK
- Gluten-Free Muffins - Page 78
- Greek Spanakopita - Page 42
- Mediterranean Sunkissed Granola - Page 47
- Lentil Salad - Page 107
- Mediterranean Quiche - Page 110
- Polenta Pizza - Page 82
- Quinoa Salad - Page 76
- Roasted Vegetable and Quinoa Bowl - Page 32
- Spanish Frittata - Page 39

www.ingramcontent.com/pod-product-compliance
Lightning Source LLC
Chambersburg PA
CBHW082243300426
44110CB00036B/2425